A Charge Nurse's Guide

Navigating the Path of Leadership

Cathy Leary, R.N. & Scott J. Allen, Ph.D.

Center for Leader Development Press
Cleveland, Ohio
www.centerforleaderdevelopment.com

A Charge Nurse's Guide
Navigating the Path of Leadership

Center for Leader Development Press
Cleveland, Ohio
www.centerforleaderdevelopment.com
cathy@cldmail.com
scott@cldmail.com

Leary, Cathy, 1943-
Allen, Scott, 1972-

ISBN: 0-9773726-0-X
Library of Congress Control Number: 2005934073

First Printing, January 2006
Printed in USA

Cover Design: Andy Shive

Production: BookMasters, Mansfield, Ohio 44905

Acknowledgements

The authors would like to thank the following individuals for their thoughtful contribution in the form of feedback, editing and encouragement.

Jessica Allen
Lisa Aurilio, R.N.
D. Barry, R.N.
Stephen B. Becker
Weezie and Bill Bradley
Julie Byrne, R.N.
Lynn Cheslock, R.N.
L. Martin Cobb
Valerie L. DeCamp, R.N.
Lisa Deptowicz, R.N.
Martha Duffy, R.N.
Nancy Haas, R.N.
Cathy L. Hadley-Samia, R.N.
Debbie Hawk, R.N.
Antoinette Kelley, R.N.
Unhee Kim, R.N.
Curtis Leary
Suzanne M. Gill, R.N.
Sarah McManus, R.N.
Thomas C. Olver
Cam Ray, R.N.
Evelyn C. Samples, R.N.
Denise Saraviti, R.N.
Lee Ann Schaffert, R.N.
Andy Shive
Amelia Smith, R.N.

<u>Dedications</u>

Cathy:

To my husband, Curtis Leary, whose love and generous spirit
sustain me.

Scott:

To my wife Jessica.

"Love does not consist in gazing at each other but in looking
together in the same direction."
—Antoine de Saint-Exupery

To all nurses everywhere.

Just before his death in 1963, the great American poet Robert Frost wrote his last poem to his nurse, Janet Forbes:

"I met you on a cloudy and dark day and when you smiled and spoke the room was filled with sunshine. The way you smiled at me has given my heart a change of mood and saved some part of a day I had rued."

A Charge Nurse's Guide

Navigating the Path of Leadership

Table of Contents

Chapter One
Me? A Leader?

Yes! You! A leader! As a charge nurse, you are in a key role to make health care work for everyone — patients, families, physicians, nurses and all the many other people who are involved in the care and healing of patients. The word that may be unexpected is *leader*. You probably did not sign up to be a leader when you decided to become a registered nurse. *Caregiver* might have been the descriptive word you had in mind — and that you are. Care giving is the essence of nursing; however, if you think about it, much of being an effective charge nurse has to do with being a good leader. A great charge nurse leads a healthcare team and its individuals to manage the care of patients therapeutically. Leadership is the key to molding a group of individuals into an effective team. Under great leadership, the team will perform the many tasks and responsibilities required for patient care. A good leader can transform a list of tasks into a coordinated approach to healing.

"You gain strength, courage and confidence by every experience in which you really stop to look fear in the face. You must do the thing you think you cannot do." — *Eleanor Roosevelt, author and 32nd First Lady of the United States*

A Balancing Act

A nurse must perform a skillful balancing act each day. You are responsible for many things — managing patients' medications, treatments, activities of daily living, managing information so that it is available to the right people at the right time, managing the schedules of diagnostic and treatment procedures handled by other departments to fit into the patient's day, managing the orientation of a new employee, documenting the status and care given to patients, and, of course, managing your time so that you can accomplish this and more in the hours allotted. *This balancing act is one of the most important things to learn*; it can be overwhelming and, at first, may even seem impossible. It is difficult because you are responsible not merely for one patient, but many. Nothing remains static.

Things are changing all around you — admissions, discharges, deteriorating patient status, unexpected demands and so forth. To be effective, you must depend upon your colleagues to work as a team. Often, this is the most challenging aspect of your job. Everyone is "doing their own thing." Each person has an assigned role of individual responsibilities. Some people prefer to work on their own and have little natural inclination to be part of a team.

An additional complicating factor is that some days you are in the role of leader and some days you are in the role of follower. Sometimes, you are the one asking for help from your colleagues. Other times, you are part of a team that is led by someone else.

"Leaders are people who do the right thing; managers are people who do things right. Both roles are crucial, and they differ profoundly. I often observe people in top positions doing the wrong things well." — *Warren Bennis, leadership author*

As charge nurse, you can save the day. You have the ability and responsibility to help everyone have a better day — what an exciting thought! To be a good charge nurse is an awesome thing. If you fully embrace this role, it is certain to be one of the greatest things you ever do.

"Leadership should be born out of the understanding of the needs of those who will be affected by it." — *Marion Anderson, contralto vocalist*

A Difficult Role

If you have served as a charge nurse before, you know there are many days when you go home thinking, "What a difficult job. This is too much for me." That is a natural feeling. Let it come and go. Your role is to meet the needs of people and the needs of people are insatiable. You simply cannot do everything for every person. Since you have chosen to be a nurse, you likely have a natural need and desire to do just that. However, after a while, it is part of what causes nurses to feel fatigued and "burnt out." Few professions are as demanding and difficult as nursing; however, it is also the noblest of professions. *You make a wonderful difference in the lives of others every day.* Remember that when you have a discouraging thought. It will help you to keep returning to your true mission. You must keep replenishing the well from which you draw each day.

"The only real training for leadership is leadership."
— *Anthony Jay, leadership author*

People and Systems

In your role as charge nurse, it is your assignment to manage the work systems and processes of the healthcare organization on behalf of the patients. The most precious asset of the healthcare organization is the people who work there. Every hand, heart and mind is required to accomplish what needs to be done. An effective charge nurse is the key to joining these two ingredients – the people and the work systems.

"We are not independent, but interdependent." — *Buddha, spiritual leader, 560-480 BC*

Sometimes the role of charge nurse is assigned to nurses who are not adequately prepared. There is usually an orientation period that consists largely of an apprenticeship or mentoring relationship in which a nurse learning the role is co-assigned to a seasoned charge nurse for a short time. In addition, there may be classes available that are helpful. These courses are usually taught at intervals during the year. However, they may or may not be convenient for a nurse to attend. Therefore, a new charge nurse may feel overwhelmed and under-prepared.

The truth is, of course, that you learn a lot on the job. While scary and even a little risky, this is a very effective way to learn. There are no classes and no mentoring that could ever fully prepare you for any given day as charge nurse because every day and every patient is different. No matter how long you serve in this role, you will learn new things as you go along. You will be amazed at how often you are faced with new challenges. The most effective approach is to get a firm grip on the basics, and your confidence will grow as you go along. A nurse is in a unique position to understand how the systems and departments of a healthcare organization work. Coupled with your growing knowledge of the individuals who manage or work in these systems and departments, this knowledge is the ticket to navigating through any situation — no matter how unusual, emergent or impossible it may seem.

"Effective leadership is putting first things first. Effective management is discipline, carrying it out." — *Stephen Covey, leadership author*

Using Your Resources

It is assumed that your clinical knowledge, patient assessment ability, capability to rescue patients in emergent situations and ability to help physicians at the bedside are solidly in place. A component of being a charge nurse is being a resource for the clinical aspects of nursing care in addition to carrying out the leadership aspects. This statement may be daunting because nurses are often thrown into the charge nurse role fairly early in their nursing careers. However, it is rare for nurses to feel they are "ready" to be in charge. This has to do with the inherent humility of new nurses as well as the fact that the role of a nurse is one of lifelong learning. You never know it all. If you are assigned to learn the role of charge nurse, embrace it, go for it. Someone thinks you are ready, even if you don't. Chances are you will thrive in the role. Never forget that you are surrounded by people who can help you; however, that does not mean that every day you should say, "I need help. I can't do all this work." It means that when you are in the rare situation of feeling as though your back is against the wall, you can reach out and ask for a hand. People usually feel good about helping one another. Get in the habit of helping others and they will be delighted to help you when you ask for assistance.

"Most U.S. corporations today are over managed and under led." — *John P. Kotter, leadership author*

Leading the Team

Being a "people person" is one of the most important assets you can bring to the role of charge nurse. Most nurses are naturally "people oriented" and like being around others. They like having fun with their co-workers. They have an optimistic philosophy about working together. They treasure the feeling that they accomplish goals as a team. *Remembering this and displaying true appreciation toward others for the unique gift that each individual brings to the patient care team is a large part of being an effective charge nurse.* This notion can rarely be taught. It is something within, which you must call forward to be the best in your role as team leader.

This book is designed to help you be a better charge nurse. It is full of ideas and tips on how to be a better leader. The authors are experienced in healthcare operations and development. Cathy has provided examples from her own experience as a nurse. Scott has provided information and resources from the field of leadership and organization development. We hope it will be useful to you and provide you with things to think about as you develop your own style and approach to the role of charge nurse.

If you embrace this challenge and give it your best shot, you will be amazed at the results. Being an effective charge nurse requires you to use your intelligence, knowledge, patience, organizational skills, emotions and people skills. You will accomplish more than you ever thought possible, and you will feel fulfilled, frustrated, tired and elated. Better than any paycheck (almost!) will be the day when, at the end of a shift, someone says to you, "The day always goes better when you are in charge."

"Not everyone can be good at both leading and managing. Some people have the capacity to become excellent managers but not strong leaders. Others have great leadership potential but have great difficulty becoming strong managers. Smart companies value both kinds of people and work hard to make them a part of the team." — *John P. Kotter, leadership author*

Reflections

Reflect on your favorite supervisor:
- What are the qualities that make this person a great leader?
- What specific traits help this supervisor connect with others?
- Which of the quotes in this chapter would best describe this person's approach to work?

Reflect upon your thoughts of being in a leadership role:
- What strengths and potential areas of weakness do you recognize in yourself? How will you manage personal areas that need improvement?
- What excites you about the charge nurse role?
- What worries you about this role?
- What articles might you read to learn more? What classes could you take?
- What individuals can you rely on for positive and constructive feedback?
- What does your supervisor expect of you?

Terms and Acronyms

- **Barriers/Roadblocks** — You face a number of barriers each day. These are problems that stop you from doing your job successfully. They often arise from communication problems or inadequate systems. Part of your job is to recognize these barriers and roadblocks and do your best to remove them for the team.
- **Leadership** — Influencing a group of people toward a common goal.
- **Management** — The act or art of managing; the manner of treating, directing, carrying on, or using for a purpose; conduct; administration; guidance; control; as, the management of a family or farm (*Webster's Revised Unabridged Dictionary*).
- **Multi-tasking** — Having many balls in the air at one time! As your responsibility in the organization increases so does the complexity of your work. Doctors, patients, co-workers, supervisors, and others will look to you to keep several balls in the air at one time.
- **System** — The *American Heritage Dictionary* defines *system* as "a group of interacting, interrelated, or interdependent elements forming a complex whole." We are all surrounded by systems every day. Restaurants have a system for getting your food to you in a timely manner. Likewise, your medical center has a system for efficiently admitting, treating, and discharging patients. When patient care is not efficient or when your fries are cold when they arrive, there is a systems problem. Finding and eliminating the root of systems problems is a part of your job.

Questions for Your Supervisor

- What do I need to know about working for you? What are your expectations?

- How will you define success in this role? What goals should I have?
- What are the five most important things on which I should focus?
- How should I approach my new role with other team members on the unit/in the department?
- Are there any special skills I need to perform my job? Based on what you know of me, do you feel there is anything I need to improve to be effective? Are there classes I can take to learn new skills?
- What will my probationary period entail? How long will it be? Who will be my mentor? How often will I get feedback on my performance?
- What are our unit goals? What is my role in helping us achieve these?
- What competencies/requirements do we have on file for team members on this unit/in this department?
- What are the traits/behaviors of successful charge nurses on this unit?

Remember...

- As a charge nurse, you are in a key role to make health care work for everyone — patients, families, physicians, nurses and all the many other people who are involved in the care and healing of patients.
- An effective charge nurse successfully manages people *and* work systems. A charge nurse plays one of the most important roles in a healthcare organization.
- There are no classes or mentoring that could fully prepare you for any given day as charge nurse because every day and every patient is different. No matter how long you serve in this role, you will learn new things as you go.
- Reflect often. Adults grow and learn through reflection. How did you do today? What could you have done better? When you stop asking these questions, you stop growing.

- Be sure you and your supervisor are on the same page. Asking the questions listed in this chapter may help you.
- You will feel fulfilled, frustrated, tired and elated. Better than any paycheck (almost!) will be the day when, at the end of the shift, someone says to you, "The day always goes better when you are in charge."

Chapter Two
Leadership

Leadership...what does it mean? Well, if you are assigned to the role of charge nurse, it means that you have responsibility for leading a team. The people you lead are not following because you are their boss or supervisor; they are taking direction from you because, when you are assigned to the role of charge nurse, they are automatically assigned to the roles of followers. The relationship between you and your peers changes with the assignment given to the work team by your supervisor or boss. There are probably days when you are a follower and someone else is the charge nurse or leader. It can be a challenge to assume this mantel of leadership without thinking through the implications of assigned or delegated leadership and the ways to carry out your role effectively.

To be effective as a leader, you must have some measure of power and influence. In fact, the first definition of *power* in the dictionary is "the ability or capacity to act or perform effectively." It doesn't mention the organizational chart and who reports to whom. It doesn't mention mandates or control. True leaders are rare and wonderful. As a charge nurse you have the opportunity to be a true leader.

"Nearly all men can stand adversity, but if you want to test a man's character, give him power." — *Abraham Lincoln, 16th President of the United States*

Leadership Styles

All of us can think of examples of good leaders and bad leaders. The most effective kind of leader may or may not be in the traditional supervisor's position. The effectiveness of good leaders has more to do with the kind of people they are rather than their titles. *Effective leaders earn the power to lead through the ways in which they relate to others.* It is truly a case of living out the Golden Rule — "do unto others as you would have them do unto you."

Coercive power tends to increase resistance of followers, whereas persuasive power tends to increase voluntary acceptance by the followers. True leaders earn their power through the enthusiastic support of their followers. People like to follow a true leader.

"All leaders are actual or potential power holders, but not all power holders are leaders." — *James MacGregor Burns, leadership author*

Most of what is said in this chapter is either common sense or knowledge you have already acquired through life's lessons. If asked to list the characteristics of an effective leader, you would come up with an excellent profile. You know the components of good leadership. The challenge is to incorporate these into your daily practice.

As a charge nurse, you will sometimes find it difficult to maintain professional and appropriate behavior. There will be interruptions and unplanned events that are disruptive to the work plan that you are attempting to accomplish. You will feel stressed and hurried. In these moments, it is easy to forget the "right" way to act and, instead, react to disconcerting circumstances in a way that diminishes your power and effectiveness as a leader.

It is a good idea to maintain an appropriate demeanor at all times. One technique is to imagine that you are in a play and the character you are playing always behaves in a positive, professional manner. When you are new at leadership this approach may help you to distance yourself a bit from personally disconcerting circumstances. It may help you to remember how to "act" until it becomes second nature. However, this approach may not work for you. Perhaps another technique will be more helpful. Give it some thought.

"Related to leadership is the concept of power; the potential to influence. There are two kinds of power: position and personal." — *Peter Northouse, leadership author*

Reflection

Even if you can recite the traits of a good leader and are effective in the charge nurse role, it is a good idea to give some thought to what makes a good leader. Reviewing the desired behaviors and thinking about *why* they work will help you to be more effective. As mentioned in the previous chapter, at the end of a shift or tour of duty, it is a good habit to review the day and think about what went well, what did not, and the effect *your* leadership had in producing these outcomes. What did you do that was effective? What did you do that was ineffective? What did you do that had a positive effect on the care of the patients? What did you do to promote teamwork? What did you do to bring out the best in each individual? What would you do and say differently, and why?

Once when I was doing rounds on the night shift, a new charge nurse said to me, "Do we have a policy that mandates people to respect the charge nurse? I don't think these people respect me, and I want to show them in writing where it says that they have to because I am in charge." I understood what she meant. I have been there. Taking charge on the night shift can be pretty difficult and lonely, especially when you have relatively short tenure and it feels like everyone else on duty has been working this shift for many years. If the new charge nurse assumes the demeanor of dictator, it turns into an unfortunate situation and every one hunkers down to watch her flounder. I am sure you have seen this play out. This happens, in part, because the charge nurse is unsure of her role. She is a little frightened and is thinking more about herself than about how the team is doing. She has likely forgotten how it feels to be a follower or member of the team.

"In organizations, real power and energy is generated through relationships. The patterns of relationships and the capacities to form them are more important than tasks, functions, roles, and positions." – *Meg Wheatley, leadership author*

Servant Leadership

It may be helpful to become familiar with the work of Robert K. Greenleaf, who has written on the concept of *servant leadership*. This philosophy fits quite naturally into the work of nurses. Nurses have chosen a profession of service. They understand what it means to serve others. In their daily work however, nurses are also called upon to lead. It is an easy shift in thinking for them to grasp the concept of a leader as the servant of the followers. The servant leader acts as a guide for a team. Likewise, the charge nurse guides the healthcare team to accomplish all that needs to be done by serving the needs of the team. Although it may seem subtle and vague at first, servant leadership is far more effective than a top-down coercive style.

Effective charge nurses are already known by peers as good team members, trusted colleagues and hard workers and they are respectful of others. They have earned the respect of peers in the role of followers. Trust and respect are components of effective leadership. Respect must be *earned*, and it starts by respecting others. Once you have earned respect, teammates grant you the power needed to lead effectively; therefore, the seeds for being an effective charge nurse have already been sown by the time you assume the role.

"You gain credibility and authority in your career by demonstrating your capacity to take other people's problems off their shoulders and give them back solutions." — *Ronald Heifetz, leadership author*

Leadership Traits

Leadership is complex. It requires you to be balanced, strong, kind and positive. It works best when you care deeply about the patients and those who care for the patients. Leadership is a big job, and it is a wonderful, fulfilling job. One of the most important behaviors you can contribute to the work of the team is your optimism and your willingness to provide positive feedback and affirmation. This communicates to the team and its members that you trust and believe in them. Optimism and a positive outlook works like a magic potion and bring out the best in everyone.

Another valuable attribute is to keep your sense of humor and find time to have some fun during your shift. This communicates a sense of well-being and acceptance that can get everyone through even the most trying of times.

When you list the attributes of a good leader, you begin to realize that there is complexity and balance involved. The leader may change behavior or demeanor depending upon circumstances or priorities. Here are some examples.

- Patient's advocate vs. physician's partner vs. peer's resource
- Firm and business-like vs. warm and friendly
- Approachable and available vs. busy and involved
- Empathetic vs. emphatic
- Being calm vs. acting quickly in emergencies
- Objective vs. subjective
- Having time vs. unavailable
- Being fair and consistent vs. seemingly unfair and arbitrary
- Engaged in team work vs. engaged in management work
- Managing by fact vs. managing by gut-feeling
- Communicating vs. thinking
- Making appropriate decisions vs. making popular decisions
- Staying on track vs. changing priorities

- Expecting a lot from oneself vs. expecting a lot from others
- Being serious vs. laughing
- ALWAYS BEING RESPECTFUL OF OTHERS

True leadership is a valuable asset of the organization. It is this heroic quality of personal engagement in the work of the organization that fulfills the mission. True leadership is also what brings you closer to self-actualization. How fortunate you are to have this opportunity.

"Leaders stand up for their beliefs and practice what they preach. They show others by their own example that they live by the values they profess. Leaders know that while their position gives them authority, their behavior earns them respect. It is consistency between words and actions that builds a leader's respect." — *Kouzes and Posner, leadership authors*

Terms & Acronyms

- **Accountability** — The act of holding someone responsible for behaviors or standards.
- **Formal Power** — An appointed position or formal authority, similar to that of your boss. Power and authority come with the position.
- **Informal Power** — Power gained without need of a formal title or position. For instance, think of the person on your unit who everyone looks to even when they are not in charge. This kind of power can be either positive or negative.
- **Influence** — *The American Heritage Dictionary* defines influence as "a power affecting a person, thing, or course of events, especially one that operates without any direct or apparent effort." You will need to use your influence to remove barriers to improve the efficiency of the systems in your place of work.

- **Reward** — The act of recognizing people when their behaviors are consistent with organizational/departmental values or standards.

Questions for Your Supervisor or Mentor

- How have other charge nurses gained respect on this unit?
- What should I work on to be among those ranks?
- What hurdles will I face along the way?
- What five behaviors do I need to exhibit in this role?
- Would you be willing to provide me with feedback along the way?
- Who on this unit can I learn from about these issues? Who is doing it right?

Reflections

- Who are the positive informal leaders on your unit?
  - How did they gain their power? Knowledge? Experience? Kindness? Consistency? Authority? Trustworthiness? Dependability? Fairness?
- What do you need to do to gain the respect of your peers?
  - Which of your behaviors need to change to meet this goal?
  - Who can help you make these changes?
- What do you need to do to meet the expectations of your supervisor?
- What is the difference between power and influence?

Remember...

- If you can master the skill of leading where you have no formal authority over those with whom you are working, research would show (Avolio, 1999) that you are well on your way to becoming an effective leader. Individuals who have the ability to influence others without the use of power have a great skill.

- The combination of skills needed to influence others varies from person to person. Think of someone in your life who has a great deal of power and influence. At times, this comes from their knowledge, extroversion, force, ability to model the way, humor, strong moral compass or work ethic. Any combination of these will serve an individual well.

- Remember that reflection and self-awareness are important for individual development and growth. If you are not honest with yourself about areas that need to improve, you will stay where you are. Clinical nurses who want to improve their skills must be honest about their deficiencies and consciously work to improve. Developing nursing leadership skills is no different. It is difficult to take a hard look at yourself and admit the need to change, but if you do, you will become stronger and better in your role as charge nurse.

Additional Resources

- *The 21 Irrefutable Laws of Leadership* by John Maxwell
- *Leadership and the One Minute Manager: Increasing Effectiveness Through Situational Leadership* by Ken Blanchard & Patricia Zigarmi
- *Who Moved My Cheese? An Amazing Way to Deal with Change in Your Work and in Your Life* by Spencer Johnson

References

Avolio, B. (1999). *Full leadership development*. Thousand Oaks, CA: Sage.

Greenleaf, R. (1977). *Servant leadership: A journey into the nature of legitimate power and greatness.* New York: Paulist Press.

Chapter Three
Self-Awareness

"Know thyself." — *Socrates, Greek philosopher, 470-399 BC*

Who are you? Who do other people think you are? It is important to consider these questions. Your ability to lead and influence others will be maximized if you are more fully self-aware. Communication with others will be more effective and powerful if you are in touch with:

- how you see yourself
- how you see others
- how others see you

There are several dimensions of awareness. First, there is who you are fundamentally — the spot where you feel at ease and in harmony within yourself; the spot where your inner thoughts and your outer actions are aligned. Second, there is who you wish you were, and may sometimes pretend to be. There is who you are on a bad day, on a good day, in an uncomfortable moment, etc. The greater your self-awareness, the less frequent the divergence from your fundamental self and, therefore, the less frequent your feelings of discomfort, anger, guilt and unease.

"I think self-awareness is probably the most important thing towards being a champion." — *Billie Jean King, tennis pro*

Of course, no matter what you do with your life, it is important to explore the concept of self-awareness. *Registered nurses are thrust into a societal role that puts them at great risk, for both poor self-esteem and ineffective performance, if they are not "self-aware."* The reasons for this are many, but they can be placed into three general categories.

1. The nursing profession attracts people who want to help others. This is good; however, there is a pathological or adverse side to wanting to help others. It is called being an enabler. The personality traits of an enabler are being over-responsible, placatory, self-critical, victimized and unconsciously worsening the problems of others. Some nurses are enablers and have issues with self-esteem. Communication coming from enablers is not always straightforward. This further complicates an already complex environment.

2. Although society recognizes nurses as professionals, they do not have all of the benefits (or risks) that society would generally recognize as being in the domain of a professional. Nurses actually function somewhere between a "blue-collar" and a "white-collar" world, which can cause conflict. Sometimes nurses *act* as professionals and sometimes they do not. This is often dictated by the circumstance in which they find themselves. Moreover, sometimes nurses are *treated* as professionals, and sometimes they are not. For example, in our society, professionals are usually not paid by the hour and they are not required to request permission to work overtime to complete the work they may be doing for a client. On the other hand, they are expected to complete the work at hand without additional pay.

3. Nurses work in a stressful, exacting, demanding, highly-charged environment. A nurse's work is not done in isolation and its very nature requires intense interaction with many people. It is inevitable that there will be conflicting priorities, verbal demands, strong emotions, ethical dilemmas and criticism.

These factors are inherent in the environment in which nurses find themselves. It is helpful to be aware of these variables. Self-awareness will help you cope and even thrive in a complex environment. You are not able to control the way that people speak and act toward you, but you *can* control the way *you* speak and act. Appropriate messages and actions on your part will have a profound effect on taking the emotion out of a situation and making communication more calm and professional. Best of all, the *patient* will remain the focus instead of the conflict among caregivers. *This is a charge nurse's goal — to keep the focus on the patient at all times.*

"Explore thyself. Herein are demanded the eye and the nerve."
— *Henry David Thoreau, author, poet, philosopher*

"Resolve to find thyself, and to know who finds himself, loses his misery." — *Matthew Arnold, poet and literary critic*

"Blessed are those who can laugh at themselves, for they shall never cease to be amused." — *Anonymous*

Choose Your Responses

In 1967, Thomas Harris wrote a book entitled *I'm OK – You're OK*. It discusses our relationships and interactions in terms of how we view ourselves. He describes three basic scenarios: *I'm not OK-You're OK*, *I'm OK-You're not OK*, and *I'm OK-You're OK*. The concept is easy to understand and very helpful in learning about oneself.

The concept makes you really think about what internal triggers cause you to react and respond in the way you do. The environment in which charge nurses work is fraught with triggers. Thinking through what makes you communicate in an ineffective or destructive manner is essential if you are to be an effective charge nurse. Then you can identify and control these triggers and *choose* your response: to act rather than react.

More recent works that expand on the topic of self-awareness as it relates to leadership are:

- *Emotional Intelligence* by Daniel Goleman
- *Primal Leadership* by Daniel Goleman, Richard Boyatzis and Annie McKee

Something happened to me when I was very new in the role of charge nurse that illustrates an interaction with the potential to cause me to say and do the wrong thing. I approached a physician when he was on the unit to see a particular patient. I stated that the nurse providing direct care to the patient had asked if the doctor could write a certain order. The physician put his face close to mine and said in a very loud voice, "Do I look like an *Attending* to you? I am a Consultant!" Fortunately, he turned on his heel and walked off the unit. There was no time for me to speak. In this case I found humor in his response to my question; however, laughing would have been as destructive as spouting off, which might have been another reaction.

Many people who write about leadership talk about *taking your time* before responding to any communication that evokes an emotional reaction in you. Take a deep breath and think about what you are about to say. A few seconds of reflection are usually all you need to become aware of your feelings. Then you are much more likely to respond in a positive or constructive way; between stimulus and response, you have the ability to *choose your response*. Doing so moves you from the position of victim to one of self-determination. Beginning your response with "I" or "The patient" usually brings forth a more assertive (rather than passive or aggressive) statement than beginning your response with, "You."

"Researchers have shown that even more than IQ, your emotional awareness and abilities to handle feelings will determine your success and happiness in all walks of life, including family relationships." — *John Gottman, author of Raising an Emotionally Intelligent Child*

Criticism Is a Gift

Criticism is something you must learn to accept. As a charge nurse, you will benefit from reflecting on how you react to criticism. Why? Everyone in a leadership role receives criticism. One of the steps toward becoming self-aware is understanding how others perceive you. Sometimes you do not present yourself as you think you do. It is helpful to know this. Learning how to accept criticism is one way to obtain this information. People find it difficult to give constructive feedback to one another. Therefore, because the messenger is anxious, it is often delivered in a hurtful or abrupt manner. If you are able to filter the facts and helpful hints from the delivery style, criticism can be a gift. Try to think of criticism like a reflection in the mirror. Use it to grow and learn; to become better. Incorporate what you have learned into your leadership style and learn how to provide others with feedback in a positive and constructive manner.

"The one important thing I have learned over the years is the difference between taking one's work seriously and taking one's self seriously. The first is imperative and the second is disastrous." — *Dame Margot Fonteyn, British ballerina*

One of the lessons I learned about self-awareness was taught to me by an elderly patient in the middle of the night. That evening, I felt there was too much to do and not enough time. Most inconveniently, the patient put on his call light. When I went to his room my non-verbal behavior must have been screaming, "I don't have time for this." He took one look at me and said, "Never mind, I'll save my question for someone else. I can see you are in too much of a rush to be a good nurse." Ouch! This incident occurred more than 20 years ago, but I will never forget the lesson.

Self-awareness is work that is never completed. It is a good idea to work on your self-awareness every day. Develop the habit of reflecting upon the events of the day. Think about how you reacted and why. This practice creates a path to self-actualization and the development of your potential as a person. It is important to like yourself and to have positive self-esteem. The more self-awareness you have the more you will like yourself. Self-awareness leads to alignment of verbal and non-verbal behavior and quiets the struggle between your internal voice and your external life. *Bottom line, self-awareness makes you a much better leader.*

"The outward freedom that we shall attain will only be in exact proportion to the inward freedom to which we may have grown at a given moment. And if this is a correct view of freedom, our chief energy must be concentrated on achieving reform from within." — *Gandhi, Indian leader*

Terms & Acronyms

- **Leader** — A person who identifies problems, works with others to identify solutions and seeks answers for the betterment of the whole.
- **Self-Awareness** — "Simply put, self-awareness means having a deep understanding of one's emotions, as well as one's strengths and limitations and one's values and motives" (p. 40). — Goleman, Boyatzis & McKee, *Primal Leadership*
- **Self Management** — Self-management allows individuals to control their feelings and impulses so they "can craft an environment of trust, comfort and fairness" (p. 47). — Goleman, Boyatzis & McKee, *Primal Leadership*
- **Whiner** — A person who is a master at identifying problems and spends hours complaining about them. Whiners often do little to be part of the solution and are blind to the fact that they may be part of the problem.

Reflections

- What "buttons" take you over the edge with physicians, other departments, etc.?
- What happens when you "go over the edge"? Do you withdraw? Yell? Communicate through the issues?
- What have you done to avoid getting to the boiling point?
- How well do you control your emotions? Can others quickly see your mood? How do they respond?

- What are three things you need to do better when it comes to self-awareness?
- What are three things you need to do better when it comes to self-management?

Self-Awareness Assessment

Rank yourself using a scale from 1-5 in which "1" is *strongly disagree* and "5" is *strongly agree*, on the following questions.

- I manage my emotions well with family, friends and co-workers.
- I am aware of my buttons or triggers.
- I am aware when they are being pushed.
- I have the ability to control how I respond with my family.
- I have the ability to control how I respond with my friends.
- I have the ability to control how I respond with my co-workers.
- My moods affect the moods of others around me.
- I have the communication skills to work through most situations.
- I am a self-aware individual.

How did you score? If you scored three or less on an item, it may be an area for improvement. Think about it…

What the Experts Say — from Primal Leadership, by Goleman, Boyatzis and McKee

- "Simply put, self-awareness means having a deep understanding of one's emotions, as well as one's strengths and limitations and one's values and motives. People with strong self-awareness are realistic — neither overly self-critical nor naively hopeful. Rather, they are honest with themselves about themselves. And they are honest about themselves with others, even to the point of being able to laugh at their own foibles" (p. 40).

- "Emotional self-awareness creates leaders who are authentic, able to give advice that is genuinely in the employee's best interest rather than advice that leaves the person feeling manipulated or even attacked. And empathy means leaders listen first before reacting or giving feedback, which allows the interaction to stay on target. Good coaches, therefore, often ask themselves: Is this about my issue or goal, or theirs?" (p. 62).

- "The Self-Aware Team – A team expresses its self-awareness by being mindful of shared moods as well as of the emotions of individuals within the group. In other words, members of a self-aware team are attuned to the emotional undercurrents of individuals and the group as a whole. Since emotions are contagious, team members take their emotional cues from each other for better or for worse. If a team is unable to acknowledge an angry member's feelings that emotion can set off a chain reaction of negativity" (p. 178).

- "Without knowing what we're feeling, we're at a loss to manage those feelings. Instead, our emotions control us. That's usually fine, when it comes to positive emotions like enthusiasm and the pleasure of meeting a challenge. But no leader can afford to be controlled by negative emotions, such as frustration and rage or anxiety and panic" (p. 45).

- "All of this is critically important to emotional intelligence. Because emotions are so contagious — especially from leaders to others in the group — leaders' first tasks are the emotional equivalent of good hygiene: getting their own emotions in hand. Quite simply, leaders cannot effectively manage emotions in anyone else without first handling their own" (p. 46).

- "Similarly, leaders who can stay optimistic and upbeat, even under intense pressure, radiate the positive feelings that create resonance. By staying in control of their feelings and impulses, they craft an environment of trust, comfort and fairness. And that self-management has a trickle-down effect from the leader. No one wants to be known as a hothead when the boss consistently exudes a calm demeanor" (p. 47).

- "Self-management also enables transparency, which is not only a leadership virtue but also an organizational strength. Transparency – an authentic openness to others about one's feelings, beliefs and actions – allows integrity or the sense that a leader can be trusted" (p. 47).

Case Study – Sandy

Sandy has been a nurse for more than 20 years. She knows everything there is to know about the unit. She has spent many years in the organization, and knows all of the doctors and managers. Sandy has excellent clinical skills. Doctors and nurses respect her for this expertise.

However, when she is in charge she acts like a dictator. She is a "know-it-all" and can be condescending to those with whom she works. In her effort to run a tight ship she barks orders and is very critical of the team. Sandy seems unaware that she is disliked as a leader. No one knows how to confront her. People are afraid that if they do say something to Sandy, they will get in trouble with the nurse manager with whom she is close.

- Do you think Sandy is aware of how her co-workers feel about her?
- How will Sandy do as a leader?
- What could those around her do to help Sandy become more self-aware?
- What could Sandy do to improve teamwork so that the focus remains on the patient(s) instead of her behavior?

Remember...

- Your moods are contagious and influence those around you. If your moods are positive and upbeat, that is a good thing; however, toxic attitudes and behaviors are destructive to you and those around you.
- Leaders who have a good system for recognizing their emotions and at the same time controlling them will likely go further in an organization. Those individuals who are open to feedback from others will likely have a better interpretation of how those around them feel about them. Also, they are more likely to make changes and improvements in their behavior and demeanor.
- We all have had experiences working for, and with, people who had no idea how challenging it was to work for them. Everything was everyone else's fault and they were masters at finding those faults; however, these people drained the energy of others, were actually part of the problem, and did not have the skills to be a part of the solution. Are you this person?

Additional Resources

- *Hard Won Wisdom: More Than 50 Extraordinary Women Mentor You to Find Self-Awareness, Perspective, and Balance* by Fawn Germer
- *Don't Give It Away: A Workbook of Self-Awareness and Self-Affirmations for Young Women* by Iyanla Vanzant
- *Visualization — an Introductory Guide: Use Visualization to Improve Your Health and Develop Your Self-awareness and Creativity* by Helen Graham
- *Toxic Leadership* by Barbara Kellerman
- www.masteryofawareness.com

References

Goleman, D. (1995) *Emotional intelligence.* New York: Bantam Books.

Goleman, D., Boyatzis, R. & McKee, A. (2002). *Primal leadership: Realizing the power of emotional intelligence.* Boston, MA: Harvard Business School Press.

Harris, T. (1967). *I'm OK – You're OK.* New York: Harper & Row, Publishers, Inc.

Chapter Four
Delegation

Delegation is an essential skill for a charge nurse. At times, you must hand off the work to team members in order to get it done.

"The surest way for an executive to kill himself is to refuse to learn how, and when, and to whom to delegate work." — *J.C. Penney, entrepreneur*

Delegation comes easily to some nurses and not to others; this truth points to an interesting phenomenon in emerging leaders. Often people who find it easy to delegate are not, in the end, the best leaders. Conversely, people who, at first, find it difficult to delegate often turn out to be better leaders. To understand why this is true, it helps to reflect upon their attitudes toward team members.

Oftentimes, people who find it easy to delegate from the very beginning are interested in lightening *their* workloads and decreasing their burden of responsibility. They see the work of management as *me* vs. *them*. *I* am the boss and *they* do the work.

As true leaders develop, they go through stages of understanding their power and responsibility to delegate; they see themselves more as members of the team than as leaders of the team. They understand that everyone is busy and that adding more work to any individual is not to be done without thought and good reason. Their first response is to try to do the work themselves. This is true for several reasons. First, they are trying to spare their colleagues additional work. Second, it is the desire of true leaders to understand the job at hand, to know what is being delegated and what it takes to get it done; to "walk in the shoes of the team members." Another reason is that, because they are truly excellent at what they do, they struggle with the thought that perhaps they may be able to do things better, faster and more accurately than other members of the team.

This last thought is actually a career decision point. Some people are happier and more successful in an arena where they can perform independently. Others prefer to work in teams or groups. Which work style is most comfortable for you?

The breakthrough happens when it becomes obvious that it is not a reasonable plan to do all the work yourself. This realization comes quickly for charge nurses — within the first few hours of assuming the role. In the end, it is a leader's responsibility to delegate not only to get the work done efficiently, but to create a team, engender trust and develop the potential of each individual team member. The process of learning and applying techniques and approaches to delegation to develop a cohesive team takes longer. In fact, it is always a work in progress for a new leader.

As with most things, there is an art and a science to delegation. The *art* has to do with interpersonal communication and team-building skills. The *science* has to do with legal and licensure issues for registered nurses.

"Surround yourself with the best people you can find, delegate authority, and don't interfere." — *Ronald Reagan, 40th President of the United States*

The Art of Delegation

The need to delegate often presents itself to the charge nurse. It takes the form of necessary tasks that are not already assigned to the members of the team. The art of delegation requires that you remember to say "please" and "thank you" when you ask someone to take on extra tasks. Successful delegation will result in the team feeling strong and capable while unsuccessful delegation causes the team to feel overworked and victimized. The difference is in the art of delegation. Here are a few suggestions to incorporate into your delegation style:

- Delegate the objective, not the procedure. Outline the desired results, not the methodology. Team members may feel micromanaged or not trusted if you tell them not only what to do, but also how to do it.
- Delegate to the right person and don't always delegate to the same person. Be fair and consistent in your delegation. Keep track of how much everyone is already doing and try not to overload any one individual. Spread tasks around.
- Clarify expectations. Make sure the person to whom you are delegating understands clearly what needs to be done and how soon.
- Check to see if the person needs additional resources to complete the task.
- Ask for feedback. Checking to see how someone is doing gives you assurance that the task is getting done. If you ask in a kind manner, it lets the person know you care about their progress.
- Express gratitude to the person to whom you are delegating. Say "thank you" at the time you delegate the task and again when the task is completed or at the end of your shift.

"You can delegate authority, but not responsibility."
— *Stephen W. Comiskey, leadership author*

The Science of Delegation

Delegation is addressed in the *American Nurse's Association Code of Ethics for Nurses* (www.nursingworld.org). Once you are licensed as a registered nurse you are accountable for knowing and living by this code. The statement on delegation says, "The nurse is responsible and accountable for individual nursing practice and determines the appropriate delegation of tasks consistent with the nurse's obligation to provide optimum patient care."

This is clarified in the Nurse Practice Act of the state in which you are licensed. You need to be familiar with what it says. Your daily actions must be consistent with the *Scope of Practice* as defined in your *Nurse Practice Act* and within the *Scope of Practice of Labor and Regulatory* laws that govern your work situation. It is safe to assume that this is incorporated into the job descriptions and policies and procedures of your organization.

You must take the time to acquaint yourself with the way it is expressed in your state's *Nurse Practice Act*. Read about it. Take a continuing education course on delegation. Ask your supervisor about it. Once you are familiar with the expectations and requirements of delegation by a registered nurse, you will feel much more comfortable with the legal aspects of who you can ask to do what.

"Words have the power to destroy or heal. When words are both true and kind, they can change the world." — *Buddha, spiritual leader, 560-480 BC*

Assess Before Delegating

Be sure to clarify the process within your facility, but some general thoughts on delegation may include:

Prior to delegation, the charge nurse must assess several things. These assessments eventually become automatic or second nature, but it is good to be aware that this is what you are assessing before delegating.

1. Assessment of the patient who needs nursing care
2. Type of nursing care the patient requires
3. Complexity and frequency of the nursing care needed
4. Stability of the patient who needs nursing care
5. Review of the assessments performed by other licensed health care professionals
6. Training, ability and skill of the person whom will be performing the delegated nursing activity

7. Nature of the nursing activity being delegated
8. Availability and accessibility of resources

Delegation can also be seen as *Five Rights* — a memory trick to help you make decisions.

1. *Right task*: One that is delegable for a specific patient
2. *Right circumstance*: Appropriate patient setting, available resources and consideration of other relevant factors
3. *Right person*: The right person is delegating the right task to the right person to be performed on the right person
4. *Right direction/communication*: Clear, concise description of the task including objectives, limits and expectations
5. *Right supervision*: Appropriate monitoring, evaluation, intervention and feedback, as needed

Finally, there are three things that cannot be delegated to anyone other than another registered nurse.

1. The initial nursing assessment and any subsequent assessment that requires professional nursing knowledge, judgment and skill.
2. The determination of the nursing diagnoses, establishment of the nursing care goals, development of the nursing plan of care and evaluation of the client's progress, in relation to the plan of care.
3. Any nursing intervention which requires professional nursing knowledge, judgment and skill. Nursing judgment is the intellectual process that an RN exercises in forming an opinion and reaching a conclusion by analyzing the data.

Something happened to me early in my days as charge nurse that illustrates the need to be clear about what you can delegate to whom. A nursing assistant approached me and volunteered to start intravenous lines. She explained that she had been a phlebotomist before becoming a nursing assistant and that she was good at difficult starts. She further stated that she knew that hospital policy prevented her from performing IV starts, but she was willing to overlook that policy if I was. This was a tempting offer since it is not always easy to find someone to start IV lines when the start is tricky and the line is needed right away. From a practical point of view, it probably would have been safe and relatively painless for the patients given the nursing assistant's previous experience; however, from a professional standpoint, the offer had to be declined given the hospital policy and the state board of nursing's position statement on intravenous lines.

Delegation is an elementary act of management. Delegation must be based upon nursing judgment, state law and organizational policies. Nursing care is dynamic and responsive to the needs of the patient. It is not practical for laws, rules and policies to list all of the specific activities that a nurse may or may not perform or delegate. Another set of guiding principles to consider when you delegate are as follows:

- *Legality* — the delegated task is within the scope of practice and not prohibited by law.
- *Competency* — the delegated task maintains standards of safe practice and the person to whom the delegation is made can demonstrate and document knowledge, skills and ability.
- *Safety* — the delegated task is safe and appropriate for the patient at this time.
- *Accountability* — the person to whom the delegation is made can perform according to standards of safe care and can accept accountability for nursing actions.

Terms and Acronyms

- **Code of Conduct** — A formal statement of the values and business practices of an organization, an entity or a professional group.
- **Delegation** — Delegation occurs when a leader or manager employs the assistance of others in completing common tasks that will benefit the unit or department.

- **Productivity** — Ratio of output to input. A process of continuous improvement in the supply of quality output or services through efficient use of inputs, with emphasis on teamwork for the betterment of all.

Case Study – Vanetta

Vanetta Jackson, RN, is the charge nurse. It is a crazy day. The lab reports are late. The physicians are all arriving on the unit for rounds at the same time — right after their 7:00 a.m. staff meeting. Several new orders have been written and need to be initiated. Six discharge orders are among them. Admitting has called with five new admissions. ICU has called with a transfer. A physician is requesting assistance with the patient in room 536. There are 30 beds on the unit and all of them are occupied. It is 8:30 a.m. and time to send half of the staff on their morning breaks. On duty are:

- Carol Smith, RN — an orientee who is new to this unit, but a seasoned nurse
- Ann Davids, RN — six years experience on this unit
- Jeff Meeks, RN — agency nurse with seven years experience
- Sonja Plusek, LPN — 20 years experience on this unit
- George Leeming, NA — four years experience on this unit
- Ann Talison, NA — 25 years experience on this unit

Carol is not returning to the unit after break because she has to go to a class for orientation. The unit secretary called in sick and the staffing office cannot send anyone to cover. The ICU patient has to be transferred onto the unit ASAP because the Department of Surgery has a fresh post-op ready to go into ICU and there are no open critical care beds. Suzie Franks of Environmental Services has stopped at the desk to say she has to go help on another unit for about an hour. One patient needs to be started on intravenous antibiotics; the IV line has to be started and someone has to go to the pharmacy to get the antibiotic because the delivery system is not working. A family member is standing at the desk and wants someone to page her mother's physician. Vanetta has just been paged to come to discharge planning rounds.

- What would you do if you were Vanetta?
- Which tasks can she delegate and to whom?
- Which of these tasks should she do herself?
- How should she prioritize what needs to be done?
- Is there any way she can get more help?
- Do you have days like this?
- What does a charge nurse do to get through a day like this?

Reflections

- When someone delegates a task to you, how do you like to be approached?
- When you have completed a task, how do you like to be recognized (simple thank you, a little note, etc.)?
- What are some creative ways to follow up with people to be sure a task has been completed (ask them to touch base with you and let you know how it went, log it in a journal, etc.)?
- How do you feel about delegation? Do you feel comfortable delegating tasks to others? Why or why not?

Remember...

- People who find it easy to delegate from the very beginning may be interested in lightening their work loads and decreasing their burden of responsibility. They see the work of management as *me* vs. *them*. *I* am the boss and *they* do the work.
- Delegation is an essential skill for charge nurses. Trying to do it all on your own simply will not work.

- True leaders see themselves more as members of the team rather than leaders of the team. At times, they may need to take control but more often than not they are simply the coordinator, making sure that everything functions well.
- There is an *art* and a *science* of delegation. The *art* has to do with interpersonal communication and team-building skills. The *science* has to do with legal and licensure issues for registered nurses. Observe how others around you practice the art and the science. Mimic those who do well and avoid the techniques of those who are ineffective. Eventually, you will feel more comfortable and your own style will emerge.

Additional Delegation Resources

- *How to Delegate* by Robert Heller
- *If You Want It Done Right, You Don't Have to Do It Yourself!: The Power of Effective Delegation* by Donna M. Genett, Ph.D.
- *Empowering Employees Through Delegation* by Robert B. Nelson
- *Delegation of Nursing Care* by Patricia Kelly-Heidenthal and Maureen Marthaler
- *Making Delegation Happen: A Simple and Effective Guide to Implementing Successful Delegation* by Robert Burns

References

American Nurse's Association Code of Ethics for Nurses. Retrieved from www.nursingworld.org/ethic on February 1, 2005.

How to Delegate. Retrieved from www.getmoredone.com on March 1, 2005.

Nursing Standards & Delegation: A Guide to Ohio Board of Nursing Rules. Retrieved from www.state.oh.us/nur/ on February 15, 2005.

Chapter Five
Utilizing Your Resources

Here's some good news: You are not alone! You are surrounded by resources to help you accomplish your job as charge nurse. In fact, the charge nurse is the person who reaches out for the appropriate resources and brings them to bear on each situation — moment to moment and patient to patient.

This chapter may seem like a list of people and things. It is. There are so many resources available to you that it is helpful to list them. There will be some you think of that are not included here, which is great. The more secure you are in the realization that you are surrounded by the ways and means to do your job, the more confident you will be in doing it. Everyone and everything is there to help you. *The trick is knowing the most effective and efficient way to access what is needed.*

"Most people have no idea of the giant capacity we can immediately command when we focus all of our resources on mastering a single area of our lives." — *Tony Robbins, leadership author*

Professional & Personal Resources

One essential characteristic fits into both categories. If you are to succeed, you must become comfortable and adept at using the information systems in your facility. We have moved past the age of each person *possessing* a body of knowledge to the age of each person *accessing* knowledge and information. It is no longer necessary to know and remember everything. However, it is necessary to know how to access information and how to navigate information systems. Health care is behind the rest of the world in developing information systems but this is just a temporary phase. Soon health care information systems will become easier to use and systems will be fully integrated. Many of the systems with which we work now are slow and difficult to navigate. Accepting this as a fact of life makes it easier to deal with.

To be effective as a charge nurse you must be skilled in the use of the communication systems of your workplace. You should know how to use the paging system, the internal and external telephone systems, the emergency/coding system, etc. Everyone is "wired up," but not everyone can be accessed in the same way. Many physicians see patients in several locations and may use paging access codes that are different from those of the health care organization where you work. One of the most valuable resources at any nursing station is a telephone book, notebook, or electronic directory with this information.

There are wonderful and unsung heroes in telecommunications — use them. Get to know them. Send them a thank you note once in a while. Telecommunications people are especially helpful in a coding or emergency situation. In a way, they are the brain center of the healthcare organization. They know what is going on all over the house and exactly how to call any code. They may know how emergency resources have been allocated at any given moment, and the back-up plan.

Very early in my career, I was the charge nurse on the night shift for a busy geriatric unit. A patient arrested during the night. I called a code. Telecommunications immediately called me to say there were already two codes going in the house. There was no third code team. Although disconcerting, this information was very helpful to me. I immediately knew that help was not on the way, and that the team on our unit had to re-prioritize and handle the situation. The patient survived!

Healthcare personnel are really at their best in emergencies. Teamwork comes naturally. Everyone focuses on the patient. Responses are rapid and skillful. Resources are brought to the team. It is an awesome thing. This is the essence of what caregivers have been educated to do. After the crisis has passed, there is a strong feeling of pride and camaraderie.

Okay — back down from the emergency mindset and consider the resources at your beck and call on a "normal" tour of duty (if there is such a thing for a nurse).

"The greatest genius will never be worth much if he pretends to draw exclusively from his own resources." — *Johann Wolfgang von Goethe, author, scientist, politician*

Professional Resources

- *Supervisor* — This person's role is to provide guidance, answer questions and assist you in doing your job.
- *Nursing Team* — There to carry out your plan of action for the day.
- *Advanced Practice Nurses* — Very helpful in developing plans of care for unusual or difficult patients.
- *Staff Development* — In your work as charge nurse, you are in a position to observe how the team is doing with various aspects of care. If you see a learning need or knowledge deficit, let someone in staff development know about it.
- *Student Nurses* — Here is where idealism meets reality and the next generation of nurses originates. Be good to these people. They need you and you need them. Remember what it was like when you were a student? *Be the nurse you always wanted to be, and they will become that nurse, too.*
- *Physicians* — Your partners in care. Get to know the personal preferences of as many of them as you can. Not every doctor, even within the same specialty, wants everything done the same way. This is a challenge. Some nursing units keep this information in a notebook at the nursing station — a nightmare for risk management, but helpful in getting through the day. Know who wants to be called at home in the middle of the night. Know who wants you to call the house staff. Know who wants their patients on the teaching service. Know who wants to use

intensivists and hospitalists. Know who covers for whom. Know who has privileges to do invasive procedures on the unit. Know why each doctor is seeing each patient — attending, specialist, consultant, etc. Facilitate communication and the passing of vital information among them.

- *Telecommunications* — They know how to connect a phone in each patient's room or how to get malfunctioning communication devices to work.
- *Information Technology/Systems* — They know about information systems and technology on your unit.
- *Intravenous Lines* — Infusing fluids, medications, blood products, etc. has to be done immediately. Getting an IV line started has to be dealt with now. Know who on your unit is an expert with difficult starts. Become one. Know who to call if you need help beyond what is immediately available.
- *Medical Records* — If you do not have access to old medical records through the information system, then know how to get the old charts on hand. The physicians will need them, and so will you and other members of the team. This should happen without your intervention but if it doesn't, know what to do, whom to call.
- *Medical Staff Office* — This department has records listing who has privileges to do what, who has new or temporary privileges and may have the schedule of the teaching staff. Again, this is probably included in the electronic information to which you have access, but, just in case…

Following is a list of other departments and services that are essential to the care of the patient. One of the basic tasks of the charge nurse is to coordinate the patient's schedule, so that all of these departments can do what they have to do, but not all at the same time. It often seems to happen that when the physician comes to visit, lunch is served, the phlebotomist arrives, and the patient is off the floor in radiology. Even if all of the scheduling systems interface there are conflicts — emergencies come first, equipment breaks down, tests take longer than planned and patients are in the bathroom. This is an everyday challenge — a job that is never done

— a test of communication skills, the ability to organize and prioritize, and diplomacy.

- *Pharmacists* — They are experts on every medication, interactions between drugs and food, etc. Coordination between some medications and blood draws are part of your responsibility. Getting medications started as soon as possible after an order is written is another component of your role. Encourage pharmacists to speak directly to physicians instead of through you — a big plus if you can facilitate it.
- *Nutritional Services* — Call on them if the patient has special dietary requests or needs.
- *Central Sterile Supply and Material Services* — These people have all of the durable medical equipment and supplies you need. These services are segmented differently in every healthcare organization. Know who has what and how to get it. Help them out by clearly marking broken equipment with a brief explanation of precisely what is wrong.
- *Social Workers/Discharge Planners* — Know who is working with each patient. Close communication is required between nursing and this department to preserve the continuum of care as the patient progresses to home, rehabilitation or extended care. If you have discharge planning rounds on your unit, it is your job as charge nurse to attend or send one of your team members. This can be difficult because everyone is so busy, but it is essential. Facilitate the communication between this department and family members.
- *Radiology* — Send an extra blanket with the patient. It is often cold in that department. Determine if a nurse needs to accompany the patient. If this is the case, temporarily reallocate your staff.
- *Rehabilitation* — Get started as soon as you get the order. Delays with scheduling PT/OT/ST are sometimes the reason for longer hospital stays than necessary.
- *Laboratory* — Having blood results available when physicians make their rounds always seems to be a

difficulty. Know when early blood draws are done and what time results are available. Know whom to call if this is off schedule.

- *Environmental Services* — Know who is assigned to your unit and know how to access them. Getting rooms cleaned promptly is essential to the efficient flow of patient care. Thank them for being a valuable part of the care giving team.
- *Security* — The services of the security department may be necessary to help you manage out-of-control situations. Get to know the members of this department. Say "hello" when they make their rounds. Their role is to watch over you and make the organization safer and more secure.
- *Clinical Engineering* — You can't do a good job if your equipment isn't working. Know the procedure for reporting broken or malfunctioning clinical equipment.
- *Facilities Maintenance* — If the plumbing is broken or the thermostat is not responsive, you need the help of the people in this department. Know how to contact them and follow their procedures.
- *Risk Management* — Know how to document and handle any incident that places people or the organization at legal risk. Know how to complete incident reports. Know how to follow through on them. Learn to recognize, document and report any patient care issues that have the potential for legal risk.
- *Families/Significant Others* — Having a good relationship with family/significant others is like having more staff. Remember what it is like to have someone you care about in the hospital, and follow the Golden Rule. The trick is to comply with HIPAA guidelines, yet to be as informative as possible. As charge nurse, you may find it is your role to facilitate communication between significant others and physicians.
- *Religious/Spiritual Leaders* — Know how to access them. Know the patient's desire. This is very important and personal, and sometimes gets a lower priority in a nurse's busy day.

- *Community or External Resources* — Social workers/discharge planners will do most of this; however, you need to know when and how to contact the coroner. Of course, you may need to give or take a report to a transferring facility or a home care nurse. Be as thorough as possible in these reports. The patient will benefit.
- *Policies and Procedures* — Within these documents is just about everything you need to know. Use them; they are designed to standardize patient care, thereby increasing safety. They are also designed to keep your daily practice within the limits required by external regulatory agencies (government, JCAHO, HIPAA, OSHA, etc.) and the laws and rules that regulate the practice of nursing in the state where you are practicing.

Personal Resources

"Happiness, to me, lies in stretching, to the farthest boundaries of which we are capable, the resources of the mind and heart."
— Leo Calvin Rosten, author and political philosopher

Listed below are the resources available to answer your questions, broaden your horizons, deepen your knowledge, develop your professional interests and advance your career. Getting involved is exciting and fulfilling. You will meet some wonderful people. Volunteering to teach in-services and classes is the best way to learn something. Read as much as you can; there are many resources available to nurses. Explore. Have fun.

- *Supervisor* — Remember that people like to be asked for advice and guidance. Your supervisor has a unique perspective. Discussing your future with your supervisor will be helpful to you and will impress upon your supervisor that you are serious about your career.
- *Mentor* — The role of mentor is to help you as you learn and develop. The great thing about mentoring is that both

parties benefit. Relationships with mentors sometimes last a lifetime.

- *Human Resources* — People in the human resources department can tell you about available classes, jobs that may take your career to the next step, and tuition benefits. They can answer questions regarding opportunities or rights as an employee of the organization. Part of their role is to be an advocate for you.
- *Staff Development* — Internal educators can provide you with the schedule and content of classes, workshops, seminars, committees and other learning opportunities. They are always interested in learning from you what classes or educational offerings would be helpful to employees.
- *Classes, In-services, Seminars* — Take advantage of the education and training offered within the organization. This is an easy and inexpensive way to earn the continuing education credits needed to meet your licensure requirements.
- *Committees* — Get involved. Become part of the solution. Meet new people. Working on internal committees is a great way to enhance your job satisfaction and expand your horizons.
- *Libraries* — Most hospitals have a library and librarians. Librarians are delighted to help you. They are knowledgeable about resources and how to find them.
- *State Board of Nursing* — This is a valuable resource in many ways. Visit the web site in your state. You can learn more about the rules and regulations that guide the practice of your profession. You can get involved with committees and the formulation of policies that create the future of nursing.
- *American Nurses Credentialing Center* — Visit www.nursecredentialing.org to learn about the requirements and testing schedule for specialty certification.
- *Professional Literature* — There are many books and journals dedicated to the nursing profession, and they are available by subscription, purchase, in libraries, on-line or

from friends and colleagues. Start a journal club. Stay informed and up-to-date.

- *Professional Organizations* — Joining a nursing organization is another way to expand your horizons, meet wonderful people and get involved in the bigger picture. There are usually several benefits to membership — journal subscriptions, reduced conference fees, online newsletters, etc.
- *The Internet* — The world is literally at your fingertips!
- *Your Personal Mission Statement* — Take the time to write your values and goals (see Chapter 12). What is important to you? Who do you want to be? Where do you want your life to go? It is surprising how much this little exercise helps in the daily journey toward self-actualization.

Terms & Acronyms

- **Accreditation** — The process by which an organization or an institution is recognized for meeting predetermined standards. One example is the Joint Commission on Accreditation of Health Care Organizations (JCAHO).
- **American Association of Colleges of Nursing (AACN)** — AACN's educational, research, governmental advocacy, data collection, publications and other programs establish quality standards for undergraduate and graduate degree nursing education, assist deans and directors to implement those standards, influence the nursing profession to improve health care, and promote public support of baccalaureate and graduate education, research, and practice in nursing (www.aacn.nche.edu).
- **American Organization of Nurse Executives** (AONE) — The mission of AONE is to represent nurse leaders who improve health care. The vision of AONE is "Shaping the future of health care through innovative nursing leadership" (www.aone.aha.org).
- **American Nurses Association (ANA)** — "The American Nurses Association is the only full-service professional

organization representing the nation's 2.7 million registered nurses (RNs) through its 54 constituent member associations. The ANA advances the nursing profession by fostering high standards of nursing practice, promoting the economic and general welfare of nurses in the workplace, projecting a positive and realistic view of nursing, and lobbying the Congress and regulatory agencies on health care issues affecting nurses and the public" (www.nursingworld.org).

- **American Nurses Credentialing Center (ANCC)** — "The American Nurses Association established the ANA certification program in 1973 to provide tangible recognition of professional achievement in a defined functional or clinical area of nursing. It certifies healthcare providers, accredits educational providers, approvers, and programs, recognizes excellence in nursing and healthcare services, educates the public, and collaborates with organizations to advance the understanding of credentialing services, and supports credentialing through research, education, and consultative services. ANCC grants certification to nursing administrators, basic and advanced" (www.nursecredentialing.org).

- **ANCC Magnet Recognition Program** — "This credentialing body recognizes healthcare organizations that provide the very best in nursing care and uphold the tradition within nursing of professional nursing practice. The program is based upon quality indicators and standards of nursing practice as defined in the ANA's Scope and Standards for Nurse Administrators. Both qualitative and quantitative factors in nursing are appraised in the credentialing process" (www.nursingworld.org).

- **Electronic Medical Record (EMR)** — An electronic document that integrates all aspects of an individual's health care.

- **Evidence-Based Medicine (EBM)** — The conscientious, explicit and judicious use of current best evidence in making decisions about the care of individual patients. The practice of evidence-based medicine means integrating individual clinical expertise with the best available external clinical evidence from systematic research.

- **Evidence-Based Nursing (EBN) or Evidence-Based Practice (EBP)** — A problem solving approach to clinical practice that integrates the conscientious use of best evidence in combination with a clinician's expertise as well as patient preferences and values to make decisions about the type of care to provide.

- **Hospitalist** — A doctor who takes care of patients when they are in the hospital. The hospitalist takes over for the primary care doctor while the patient is in the hospital, keeps the primary care physician informed of the patient's condition and progress, and turns the care of the patient back to the primary care physician when the patient is discharged from the hospital.

- **Human Resources** — Defined by the *American Heritage Dictionary* as "the persons employed in a business or organization; personnel."

- **Human Resources Department** — The people who serve as liaison for all personnel who work in organizations.

- **Intensivist** — A board-certified physician who is additionally certified in the subspecialty of critical care medicine.

- **Joint Commission on Accreditation of Healthcare Organizations (JCAHO)** —The mission of JCAHO is "To continuously improve the safety and quality of care provided to the public through the provision of health care accreditation and related services that support performance improvement in health care organizations" (www.jcaho.org).

- **Legislative Network for Nurses** — This is a newsletter from Business Publishers, Inc. that summarizes and updates policy and politics for the nursing profession (www.bpinews.com).

- **National Black Nurses Association, Inc. (NBNA)** — The NBNA mission is to provide a forum for collective action by African American nurses to "investigate, define and determine what the health care needs of African Americans are and to implement change to make available to African Americans and other minorities health care commensurate with that of the larger society" (www.nbna.org).

- **National Student Nurses' Association (NSNA)** — "The NSNA mission is to organize, represent and mentor students preparing for initial licensure as registered nurses, as well as those enrolled in baccalaureate completion programs; convey the standards and ethics of the nursing profession; promote development of the skills that students will need as responsible and accountable members of the nursing profession; advocate for high quality health care; advocate for and contribute to advances in nursing education; and develop nursing students who are prepared to lead the profession in the future" (www.nsna.org).
- **Occupational Safety & Health Administration (OSHA)** — "OSHA's mission is to assure the safety and health of America's workers by setting and enforcing standards; providing training, outreach, and education; establishing partnerships; and encouraging continual improvement in workplace safety and health" (www.osha.gov).
- **Policies and Procedures** — Written documents that detail the clinical, business, and other practices of the organization.
- **Resources** — Three definitions of the term resources according to the *American Heritage Dictionary*: something that can be used for support or help; an available supply that can be drawn on when needed; means that can be used to cope with a difficult situation.
- **Sigma Theta Tau International (STTI)** — "Sigma Theta Tau International, Honor Society of Nursing, provides leadership and scholarship in practice, education, and research to enhance the health of all people. STTI supports the learning and professional development of its members, who strive to improve nursing care worldwide" (www.nursingsociety.org).
- **The Health Insurance Portability and Accountability Act of 1996 (HIPAA)** — HIPAA disseminates and monitors compliance with national standards to protect the

privacy of personal health information. Failure to comply can result in federal penalties, compromised patient privacy, decreased consumer trust, damage to the healthcare organization's reputation, and lost reimbursement. Healthcare organizations are mandated to train, monitor, and censure employees regarding the HIPAA Standards for Privacy and Security (www.hipaa.org).

Reflections

- What resources do you have at your disposal to get your job done?
- What educational resources are offered by your organization?
- Who in your organization might serve as a mentor?
- Who in your organization will you need on your team to get things done?
- What non-human resources are at your disposal? Technology? Other tools?

Case Study — Janet

Janet's supervisor recently assigned her to the duty of charge nurse saying, "I have great faith in your technical competence and know you will be great in the role." This made Janet feel good considering she had only been a nurse for one year...and what a wild one it had been! Janet was all business when it came to getting her work done. She did not spend a lot of time gossiping or chumming around with the other nurses. To her, the patient was first, and she spent little time on anything else. It was no surprise to others on her unit when she was assigned to charge, but some were worried that she would try to rule with an iron fist and expect everyone else around her to work the same way she does. Patty, a nurse of 23 years, even went so far as to say that she would not follow Janet. She was young, naïve and "a company woman" in Patty's eyes. Others agreed.

Janet was unaware of these feelings. Her supervisor (Pam) was aware, but thought she would wait and see how things progressed in the first couple of weeks. Besides, Pam did not have a lot of time to hold Janet's hands as JCAHO was due for a visit any time. Pam had been in meetings and, so long as the floor was not on fire, she felt everything was okay.

- What are the red flags in this story?
- How will Janet effectively lead those around her?
- What are the barriers that Janet will face?
- What resources are available to Janet?

Case Study – Penny

Penny has been a charge nurse for 10 years. She loves being in charge and likes everyone with whom she works. She bends over backward to cover for others and ensure that everything runs smoothly on her watch. As a result, everything seems to be running like clockwork. She loves the fact that everyone feels comfortable coming to her with problems and she loves being part of the solution, even if it means that she needs to step in and cover.

Lately, Penny's supervisor has been on her case because she noticed that Penny is not holding co-workers accountable. To Penny, these issues are minimal and she blows them off as one time events. Penny likes being the person on whom everyone relies. Doctors are always telling her she is the best and they would be lost without her.

Pressure from her supervisor to slow down and confront inappropriate behavior has been mounting. Penny thinks it will pass. Her boss is determined to stay on her.

- What are the red flags in this story?
- How does Penny need to change?
- What are the barriers that Penny faces if she changes?
- What resources are available to Penny?

Remember...

- The charge nurse is the person who reaches out for the appropriate resources and brings them to bear on each situation — moment to moment and patient to patient.
- It is no longer necessary to know and remember everything. *However, it is necessary to know how to access information and how to navigate information systems.*
- One of the basic tasks of the charge nurse is to coordinate the patient's schedule, so all of the departments can do what they have to do to care for the patient properly.
- Getting involved is exciting and fulfilling. You will meet some wonderful people. Volunteering to teach in-services and classes is the best way to learn. Read as much as you can; there are many resources available to nurses.
- Utilize your resources. There is no need to go it alone. Not only will you be better at your job, you will save time.

Additional Resources

- *Achieving Success Through Social Capital: Tapping Hidden Resources in Your Personal and Business Networks* by Wayne E. Baker

Chapter Six
Clarifying Expectations

One day when I was the charge nurse, I asked the bedside nurse for an update on the discharge plan for one of our patients who was to go home the next day. I was dismayed when she said, "He went home an hour ago. Did you say discharge *tomorrow*!? I thought you said discharge *today*. Should I call the doctor and tell him the patient has already been discharged?"

This is not what you want to hear from a member of the team. This is the hard way to learn about the importance of clarifying expectations. Of course, this example is an extreme one in which many concepts of safe practice and nursing judgment have been violated. But it makes the point about how terribly wrong things can go when just one word is misunderstood. Communicating clearly and clarifying one another's expectations are extremely important in the care of patients and their safety. Further, it saves everyone a lot of precious time.

"The quality of our expectations determines the quality of our actions." — *Andre Godin, French socialist*

Expectations of Stakeholders

It is a good idea to think about the expectations of all parties. The first step in clarifying expectations is awareness of your stakeholders. Here is a partial list of possible stakeholders:
- patients
- significant others of the patients
- supervisor
- nursing team
- physicians
- extended team — other departments and disciplines
- organization that employs you

- partners external to the organization (e.g., home care nurses)
- external regulatory bodies (e.g., State Nursing Board, JCAHO and the Department of Health)
- you

Wow! It is a long list, and it is sobering to realize how many people depend on you to be clear in what you say and do. Looking at it another way, it is stunning to see how many people you depend upon to clarify their expectations of you. In truth, it is not as overwhelming as it seems at first, because much of it boils down to one statement: *Do what is right for the patient(s)*. This thought will always be the right one to have. Thinking of the patient as your primary reason for being there is always helpful in setting priorities and figuring out what to do.

Although doing what is right for the patient is the basic tenet or precept of a charge nurse's work, it is not so simple to figure out what *is* right for the patient. The patient, their significant others and every professional involved in the patient's care may have different opinions. Each has individual biases, unique experiences, professional education/knowledge, other pressing priorities and personal desires and motivations. As charge nurse, you must consider input from all parties. Then, acting as the patient's advocate and leader of the team, you must make the best possible decisions…quickly, which is not easy.

"A master can tell you what he expects of you. A teacher, though, awakens your own expectations." — *Patricia Neal, actress*

Expectations of Yourself

Returning to the above list, you will note that one of the stakeholders to consider is you. To keep the patient at the top of the list, you must first understand yourself. Therefore, it is a good idea to clarify the expectations you have for yourself. Your expectations probably include: giving the best care possible to each patient, having a collegial relationship with your peers, improving and learning each day, having fun, being a role model, impressing your supervisor, being strong, feeling fulfilled, knowing you are making a positive difference in the lives of others, being trusted and respected, and being accountable and responsible. Reflecting upon what you expect from yourself is a good exercise. Doing so keeps you grounded in a deep understanding of the greater meaning of your work. It helps you to keep growing and learning.

Conversations with your supervisor are very important. Sometimes you have to arrange them. Don't hesitate to request a meeting if one is not scheduled. You deserve to find out how you are doing from the supervisor's perspective and the supervisor owes it to you. You will learn what is expected of you through your position description, orientation, competency testing, in-services and policies and procedures; but especially your peers, mentors and supervisors. Ask what you are doing right. Ask what aspects of your practice need improvement. See how the responses fit with your self-expectations. This reflective process will make you a better charge nurse.

Ultimately, you will feel as though you are part of the "bigger picture" if you know what the organization expects of you. What is the mission statement? What is the strategic plan? What action plans are applicable to your nursing unit? What things are being measured by the performance improvement/quality assurance/total quality management department? How does your daily practice help achieve these goals?

"Winners make a habit of manufacturing their own positive expectations in advance of the event." — *Brian Tracy, leadership author*

Communicate to Clarify Expectations

The nitty-gritty of nursing practice rests in the communication and clarification of expectations with patients, significant others and physicians. As you know, clarifying expectations is not as easy as it sounds because many factors implicit to healthcare have a negative effect on the clarity and thoroughness of communication. Be aware of them. Factors include: stress, frustration, anxiety, anger, pain, illness and multi-tasking. It takes time to clarify expectations with each other, but it saves time in the end...and it is much more therapeutic for the patient.

It is always a good idea to remember that if people do not know what is expected of them, there is no way to hold them accountable for their actions or lack of actions.

"Set your expectations high; find men and women whose integrity and values you respect; get their agreement on a course of action; and give them your ultimate trust." — *John Akers, former IBM chairman*

In your role as charge nurse you need to clarify expectations many times each day. Speak clearly. State the facts. In a kind way, ask people if they understand what you've said. Listen to their responses. If there is confusion or disagreement, stop. Discuss things until there is consensus. Listen to the other person's point of view. Stephen Covey's fifth principle in *The 7 Habits of Highly Effective People* is: "Seek first to understand, then to be understood." If you are taking directives from someone else (e.g., orders from a physician), repeat them. Ask questions if there are confusing or conflicting messages. Make sure expectations are clarified. As you know, this is sometimes difficult if the messenger is in a hurry or in an impatient state of mind; however, as the patient's advocate, you have to work through these barriers and clarify the expectations. In the end, it will save everyone a lot of time and the patient will get the right care. Repeating verbal orders to the initiator is not only wise and safe, but also required by JCAHO.

"If you paint in your mind a picture of bright and happy expectations, you put yourself into a condition conducive to your goal." — *Norman Vincent Peale, author and clergyman*

As the charge nurse it may be your role at times to help patients and their significant others understand things that are confusing them. This is often not an easy task, or a quick one. It requires time, listening, detective work and, sometimes, facilitating communication among members of the healthcare team. There are many people who come in and out of a patient's room and to the patient (and maybe even to you) they do not all seem to be on the same page. If there are several physicians on the case, they may not be aware of what each other has said to the patient. The same is true of other caregivers. It gets even more complicated when there are several significant others who have heard mixed messages and perceive the situation in different ways. Trying your best to clarify expectations in these situations is critical. The results of patient satisfaction surveys always show that what patients want most is information and communication. So even if it takes a long time and is difficult to do, it is worth it — well worth it — to listen to the questions and concerns of the patient and family and then to clarify, as much as you can, what the patient can expect from the healthcare team. You and your nursing team are the people closest to, and most trusted by, the patient. The positive effect you have in communicating with the patient goes a long way toward promoting healing and giving the patient a sense of well-being.

"Our limitations and successes will be based, most often, on our expectations for ourselves. What the mind dwells upon, the body acts upon." — *Denis Waitley, leadership author*

Terms & Acronyms

- **Performance Improvement (PI), Quality Assurance (QA), Total Quality Management (TQM)** — These are comprehensive and structured approaches that seek to improve the quality of care and services through ongoing refinements in response to continuous measurement and feedback. All of these approaches focus on improving the systems around you so that outcomes are improved. What barriers to quality care exist on your unit? What process do you use to improve systematically?

Things to Do

- Read the position description of a charge nurse for your facility.
- Know the expectations of your supervisor.
- Know the expectations of your co-workers.
- Know the expectations of the doctors.
- Know the expectations of regulatory organizations such as JCAHO.
- Know the expectations of your patients and their significant others.
- Articulate what the above mentioned people can expect from you.
- What expectations do you have for yourself in the charge nurse role?

Reflections

- Are you comfortable with the idea of clarifying the above mentioned expectations?
- If not, why? What could the ramifications be?
- What are some ways to find answers to the statements in the "Things to Do" section?
- Who among your peers does a great job of setting expectations? Why are they successful?
- What happens when clear expectations are not part of the culture? How does this affect patient care?

Case Study – County Medical Center

You are relatively new to County Medical Center (CMC) and within two years have just been assigned to be in charge on the late shift in the ICU. You work nights and often feel somewhat disconnected from the "daytime" medical center.

However, you are excited to be in this new role and want to make a difference. You have always known that your strengths lie in your people skills. You have an ability to work with people of all kinds and not get caught up in some of the "catty" aspects of the unit. You are unfamiliar with the role of charge nurse, and by no means do you have a grasp of the many administrative or managerial policies and procedures.

Although the players change each night, your team usually is comprised of the following individuals:

- Sandy Johnson, RN, MSN, has been in the ICU for 23 years. She knows everything there is to know about the ICU and is very involved; however, she is extremely overbearing and will tell *everyone* her thoughts on *everything*. She is not happy that you are the charge nurse.
- Tina Lately, RN, and Cheri O'Malley, RN, BSN, pretty much keep to themselves. They spend most of their break time together and do their jobs, but are not willing to do much beyond that. They tend to feed the rumor mill but, more often than not, they can be counted on to get their jobs done.
- Jenny Peters, RN, BSN, and David Rae, RN, have been with CMC for 12 years. Their families come first and often they arrive late because of family commitments. They are good employees, but rarely get to work on time and take frequent breaks.
- Cathy Peterson, RN, is the nicest person to be around and is very agreeable; however, her mistakes are abundant. It seems that you spend a good portion of your time cleaning up after Paula or listening to others complain about her inadequacies.

- Jessica Walters, RN, and Molly Mathers, RN, BSN, have been at odds with each other for years. They are constantly in conflict and, when not talking about each other, they are talking about how inadequate everyone else is. They each run with some of the above-mentioned individuals and often their differences boil over into the two cliques. Both Jessica and Molly like to tell others about their issues with the other. Everyone is tired of it.
- Laura Lednik, RN, Mary Tharp, RN, and Jayna Winkler, RN are your closest friends on the unit. They have stuck with you through thick and thin. They always keep you "in the loop." None of them is perfect and at times they gossip. They have punctuality issues but you feel strongly that they are good people and are "here for the patient."
- Wanda Wallingford is the unit secretary and has been with the organization for 30 years. She is kind, compassionate and trustworthy. She seems to be the glue that holds things together.
- Two EMTs work on your unit and both have a bit of an attitude. Martin Cobb can be lazy and always has to be told what to do. Jud Horras is very competent, but has personality conflicts with many people on the unit.

  o List five things can you do to promote teamwork on the unit?
  o What are five things you can do to improve communication on the unit?
  o What are five ways to provide feedback to your team members with performance issues? How do you set expectations with everyone?
  o What are five things you need to keep in mind as you begin working with your unit?
  o What resources/tools may assist you in providing excellent care to the patients?

Remember...

- "Take the needed time to work with individuals who are not meeting your expectations. It is important not only for you to communicate initially what you expect, but also if you see a consistent pattern that is not what you are looking for, take the time to adjust it. Don't ignore it and let it continue; if you do, you'll either be the one redoing the project or getting consistently frustrated. Managing people takes energy and part of that role is to help people be as effective as they possibly can. Of course, the desire is their responsibility; the process, though, could be part yours." — Peggy L. McNamara

- It is a good idea to clarify the expectations you have for yourself. Your expectations probably include: giving the best care possible to each patient, having a collegial relationship with your peers, improving and learning each day, having fun, being a role model, impressing your supervisor, being strong, feeling fulfilled, knowing you are making a positive difference in the lives of others, being trusted and respected and being accountable and responsible.

- In all of your interactions, remember Stephen Covey's fifth principle in *The 7 Habits of Highly Effective People*: Seek first to understand, then to be understood.

- As charge nurse, it may be your role to help patients and their significant others understand things that are confusing. Often, this is not an easy task, or a quick one. It requires time, listening, detective work and, sometimes, facilitating communication among members of the healthcare team.

Additional Resources

- *Managing Patient Expectations: The Art of Finding and Keeping Loyal Patients* by Susan Keane Baker
- *Managing Expectations* by Naomi Karten

- *Exceptional Customer Service: Going Beyond Your Good Service to Exceed the Customer's Expectation* by Lisa Ford, *et al.*

References

Covey, S. (1989). *The 7 habits of highly effective people.* New York: Simon & Schuster.

Chapter Seven
Facilitating Change

The fact that few people enjoy changes at work is curious since everything changes all the time. We change. The people around us change. The seasons change. Life is full of changes!

Many changes take place naturally. Things change without us taking much notice and certainly without our involvement or manipulation. We grow older. The trees grow taller. A favorite restaurant changes its menu.

We initiate and participate in many changes. We educate ourselves, find partners, have children and buy houses, cars and clothes. These are positive changes which we call "progress;" however, at times we are unwilling participants in changes that we perceive as negative because they are emotionally or financially draining, and because they are beyond our control. They make us feel powerless. We call these "life," as in "that's life." For example, family members lose their jobs, cars break down, etc.

In fact, there is very little that remains constant or stable in our lives. Every change requires us to regain our personal sense of balance and well-being. Depending on the effect of the change we are experiencing, the adjustment may be huge or minimal.

"They say that time changes things, but you actually have to change them yourself." — *Andy Warhol, artist*

Change is Stressful

Because change is stressful and omnipresent, we try to avoid the disruption whenever we feel that it is unnecessary or even harmful, and whenever we feel we may have the power to stop it. Each of us has only so much capacity for stress and, as we mature, we know when we are near the point of painful imbalance. If the change we face seems more like an irritant than a positive, we fight against it. Avoidance of change may work when the environment in which the change is occurring is under our control or in our personal domain.

When change is happening in our workplace it becomes more complex. Some people regard work as a place to put in a few hours to get a paycheck. There is so much going on in their personal lives that they feel they can not afford to invest a lot of extra energy or effort in their work. They are "maxed." They are victims. Change makes them feel tired, frightened, angry, stupid and/or incompetent. What they do not realize is the amount of negative energy and toxic effort they can pour into the workplace with their resistance to change. They increase their own stress and the stress levels of everyone around them. They erect barriers that slow progress. Their negativity takes the joy out of what could be a positive and hopeful learning environment.

"Change means movement. Movement means friction. Only in the frictionless vacuum of a nonexistent abstract world can movement or change occur without that abrasive friction of conflict." — *Saul Alinsky, political activist*

Coping with Change

It is human nature to react to change. Some people cope with change better than others. Understanding that everyone goes through a personal process of adjustment when faced with change is helpful.

During my orientation period as a brand-new registered nurse, a revised form was introduced that changed the way we documented the care of patients with diabetes. I remember thinking, "I am really going to like this job when they stop changing things." Little did I know. And this was back in the day when only one thing changed at a time and there was time between changes! Change is inherent in health care. It improves our ability to care for our patients. This is a good thing. The system has a lot of room for improvement. Therefore, to find the workplace personally fulfilling, a nurse must learn to embrace change. Further, to be an effective charge nurse, it is necessary to be a change agent.

"Everything changes, nothing remains without change." — *Buddha, spiritual leader, 560-480 BC*

A Theory of Change

In 1960, Everett Rogers published a study on the topic of *Diffusion of Innovation Theory*. I stumbled upon this when I was exploring the literature about change. I was trying to understand the behavior of physicians and nurses in reaction to the introduction of an electronic medical record. Mr. Rogers concluded that, when people are faced with the introduction of innovations in the workplace, they fall into five categories: *innovators, early adopters, early majority, late majority and laggards.*

Innovators and *early adopters* make up roughly 17 percent of the workforce. They embrace change and make it part of their daily routine. They understand the positive qualities and the performance improvement embedded in change. They find change compatible with their existing values, past experiences and needs. They do not find change overly complex to understand and use. They apply themselves to learning how to implement the change and they move on.

"It's not the strongest of the species that survives, nor the most intelligent. It is the one that is most adaptable to change." — *Charles Darwin, British naturalist*

The three remaining categories make up roughly 83 percent of the workforce. These people resist change. They prefer to observe others incorporating change. They watch for visible results. They need further proof that change is worth the effort. They want someone else to engage in a trial application before they invest themselves. They engage in verbal behavior that casts dispersions and doubts on innovation.

Knowing this is helpful when you are a charge nurse. Think about which category best represents you and those on your unit. You are in a key position to be a change agent. The good news about Mr. Rogers theory is that the 17 percent can have a positive and powerful effect upon the remaining 83 percent. Being a change agent is easier when you understand where everyone is coming from. You can have a positive influence on your coworkers when you understand their coping mechanisms.

"Change is the law of life. And those who look only to the past or present are certain to miss the future." — *John Fitzgerald Kennedy, 35th President of the United States*

Be a Change Agent

Being a change agent requires you to be a role model for others. Be the change. Embrace it. Be flexible, agile and positive. Keep trying until you "get it." Learn everything you can and help others to learn. Talk about the positive reasons for the change. Relate the change to *improved patient care* — this mantra is the common ground. When those who fear and resist change realize that they have a positive personal mentor, it is like having a lifeline to hold on to in deep water. The fear of incompetence or failure can be paralyzing. This is dangerous in the arena of patient care. When people are placing negative energy into resisting change, they are not placing positive energy into patient care. They are concentrating on the wrong thing. They are thinking more about themselves than the patients.

"God grant me the serenity to accept the things I cannot change, the courage to change the things I can, and the wisdom to know the difference." — *Reinhold Niebuhr, theologian*

Approach the adoption of change as a team. Teams are stronger than individuals. Be supportive of one another. Openly discussing the effect of the change is helpful, especially to those who resist it. They realize they are not alone. They hear about the approaches that have worked for others. They hear about frustrations and how they were overcome. The trick is to keep these conversations positive. Work on nurturing a positive culture that embraces change.

Become involved in committees and task forces that are developing innovations and changes. Let your supervisor know that you are interested in doing this. These work groups need the input of front-line nurses. They are always well-meaning in their attempts to improve the quality and efficiency of patient care; however, decision makers sometimes do not have the input that is essential to make innovations fit with reality. Lacking the right input, there is bound to be a gap between the planned change and the everyday reality.

"Never believe that a few caring people cannot change the world. For, indeed, that's all who ever have." — *Margaret Mead, sociologist*

Several years ago in a hospital where I was working, the first phase of using information technology in the daily nursing routine was implemented. As in most hospitals, the nurses in this facility were very dependent upon the Kardex. This was a working document relied upon by everyone to keep track of what was going on with every patient. It was sort of a current list of what needed to be done coupled with need-to-know facts about each patient. It was vital to the safety and efficiency of patient care. In the planning of electronic nursing documentation, the importance of the Kardex was minimized. Information technology staff, of course, did not understand it as they had not experienced its use. Nurses who were on the planning committee did not adequately stress its importance and function. It was so much a part of their work lives that it never occurred to them to emphasize it.

We were all very new at this. We had never experienced an actual "go-live" of anything that had a direct effect on patient care. In any case, it was devastating to the efficient flow of work when, upon implementation, it was discovered that there was no Kardex as we had known it. It was there, but it was hard to find, and it was not the living, breathing, dog-eared document that we relied upon. Case in point — get on a planning committee and make the needs of nurses known.

"If one desires a change, one must be that change before that change can take place." — *Gita Bellin, philosopher, educator, aesthetics lecturer*

Get Involved! Another reason, of course, is that if you know why certain decisions were made, it is a lot easier to explain the final product to the *late majority* and *laggards*.

"If you think you're too small to make a difference, then you haven't been in bed with a mosquito." — *Anita Roddick, founder of The Body Shop*

The Reality of Change

It is important to unscramble the *myth* of change from the *reality* of change, and to interpret it for the *late majority* and *laggards*. There is a marketing quality to the stories the frontline is told about innovations. They are told that the changes will make their work more efficient, more error free, faster and better for the patient, the nurse and the physician (and eventually they will). These messages are designed to achieve "buy-in." The problem with this spin is that it skips over the implementation phase, the learning curve, the "working-the-bumps-out" part of any change. Not only does it omit any mention of this phase but it also implies that implementation will be easy and seamless. In reality the implementation phase is often difficult. The new technology is disruptive and hard to use. Everything takes longer. Learning the new way takes place while unlearning the old. Frustration rules, tempers flare and impatience reigns. Admitting this to one another and acknowledging it as a normal part of implementing change helps one another cope. Not discussing it makes it harder to cope and causes people to doubt their own competence.

"Leaders are visionaries with a poorly developed sense of fear and no concept of the odds against them. They make the impossible happen." — *Dr. Robert Jarvik, American cardiac surgeon*

As a champion of change it is important for you to be aware that change implementation usually has two purposes: one is to *alter the manner* in which we do things — a new form, switching from pen and pencil to inputting electronically, upgrading technology, etc., and the second is to *improve our processes and outcomes.* Therefore, we are often asked to learn two new concepts, not one. In a sense, the first is mechanical and the second is cognitive. The ease of implementing changes aimed at improving patient care is directly related to the gap between the old way and the new. The larger the gap, the longer the change will take, and the harder it will be to sustain.

Being a change agent is an essential element to being the best charge nurse you can be. It also swings wide the doors for further leadership opportunities. A positive attitude, solid work ethic, profound respect for others, sound clinical competency, consistently good interpersonal relationships, exceptional communication skills, a robust sense of humor and the ability to be a change agent is the winning combination for any leadership path that you may wish to take.

"Belief at the beginning of an endeavor is the one thing that will ensure success." — *William James, psychologist and philosopher*

What the Experts Say

- "People change what they do less because they are given analysis that shifts their thinking than because they are shown a truth that influences their feelings." — John P. Kotter
- "Leadership is a relationship, founded on trust and confidence. Without trust and confidence, people don't take risks. Without risks, there's no change. Without change, organizations and movements die." — Jim Kouzes and Barry Posner
- "Whatever the challenge, all involve a change from the status quo." — Jim Kouzes and Barry Posner
- "Habits, values and attitudes, even dysfunctional ones, are part of one's identity. To change the way people see and do things is to challenge how they define themselves." — Ronald Heifetz & Marty Linsky
- "One major reason people resist organizational change is that they think they will lose something of value as a result. In these cases, because people focus on their own best interests and not on those of the total organization, resistance often results in politics or political behavior." — John P. Kotter
- "One of the most common ways to overcome resistance to change is to educate people about it beforehand. Communication of ideas helps people see the need for and the logic of a change. The education process can involve one-on-one discussions, presentations to groups or memos and reports." — John P. Kotter
- "If the initiators involve the potential resistors in some aspect of design and implementation of the change, they can often forestall resistance. With a participative change effort, the initiators listen to the people the change involves and use their advice." — John P. Kotter
- "The combination of cultures that resist change and managers who have not been taught how to create change is lethal." — John P. Kotter

Terms & Acronyms

- **Change Agent** — an individual who leads or acts as a catalyst for change in an organization, department or community.
- **Change Initiative** — an initiative with the specific purpose of changing organizational norms and behaviors.
- **Change Management** — the act of managing or controlling the process of organizational change. Change management is often associated with a plan of action designed in advance.

A Theory of Change

This is a *simple* model of change. Any time a change occurs within your family, at work or in a community group, the following four elements should be in place for the change to stick. If any one of these is not in place, it is likely that the desired change will not occur.

- <u>Behavior</u> — What are the behaviors you are hoping to change? These must be clearly defined and communicated to all involved. **Beware!** One of the biggest problems in organizations is the feeling that we have effectively communicated something when we have not.

- <u>Training</u> — This is a graphic example, but it will stick with you. If you put a gun to someone's head, could they employ the desired change? If the answer is yes, then there is not a training issue. There may be a communication or accountability problem. **Beware!** One of the biggest mistakes made by organizations is the belief that training alone will fix a problem.

- <u>Accountability</u> — Accountability is the real issue in many organizations. People have heard about the change and they could do it if they had to, but for some reason they just don't. **Beware!** Before you implement any change initiative, you must plan for a system of accountability. Failing to discuss how people will be held accountable to the new behavior is a sure way to fail.

- **<u>Reward</u>** — Reward those individuals who embody the changed behavior. This does not need to be a trip to Hawaii or anything big. A simple "thank you" will do. If accountability is the stick, then reward is the carrot. Again, before introducing change, you need to plan how you will reward people for the new behavior. **Beware!** If you do not plan for reward, people will not be as motivated to employ the new behavior.

Reflections

- What changes have you witnessed in your area?
- Of the ones that failed, what happened? Of the ones that succeeded, why? Were they successful?
- What are some of the major challenges your organization faces when implementing a change?
- What are some of the major challenges your unit faces when implementing a change?
- What are some of the major challenges *you* face when implementing a change?
- What can you do to help facilitate change on your unit?
- What challenges will you face?
- What resources can you tap to help you along?
- Who in the organization can help you along?

Case Study – Scripting

You are the charge nurse during day shift on a pediatric unit. Your supervisor has told you that administration would like you to implement *scripting*. Nurses are to use scripted messages when they speak with patients. For instance, when you are about to leave a patient's room you are to say, "Is there anything else I can do for you?" You have been told that this approach improves customer satisfaction and makes life easier for nurses. Hmmm...you do not see how this is will make your life *any* easier. There are already a million things going on.

Regardless, your supervisor asks you to implement the scripting on your shift. You know those around you will have a fit — another flavor of the month. To make it worse, you are not even sure you agree with the new request.

- How do you go about implementing this change?
- What resources are at your disposal to help in making this adjustment?
- How will your demeanor and attitude toward the change impact its successful implementation?
- What is your plan of action?

Remember...

- "Change means movement. Movement means friction. Only in the frictionless vacuum of a non-existent abstract world can movement or change occur without that abrasive friction of conflict." — Saul Alinsky
- There is very little that remains constant or stable in our lives. Every change requires us to regain our personal sense of balance and well-being.
- Everett Rogers' *Diffusion of Innovation Theory*: when people are faced with the introduction of innovations in the work place they fall into five categories: *Innovators, early adopters, early majority, late majority and laggards.*
- Behaviors, training, accountability and rewards must all be part of your plan. If they are not, it will likely fall short.
- The implementation of change usually has two purposes. The first is to *alter the manner* in which we do things — a new form, switching from pen and pencil to inputting

electronically, upgrading technology, etc. The second is to *improve our processes and outcomes*. Therefore, we are often asked to learn two new concepts, not one.

Additional Resources

- *Change Management Resource Library* — www.change-management.org
- *Who Moved My Cheese? An Amazing Way to Deal with Change in Your Work and in Your Life* by Spencer Johnson & Kenneth H. Blanchard
- *Leading Change* by John P. Kotter
- *The Heart of Change: Real-Life Stories of How People Change Their Organizations* by John P. Kotter & Dan S. Cohen
- *Change Management* by Jeffrey Hiatt & Timothy Creasey
- *The Leadership Challenge* by Jim Kouzes & Barry Posner
- *Leadership on the Line* by Ron Heifetz & Marty Linsky

References

Rogers, E. (1960). Diffusion of Innovation Theory. Retrieved from http://uts.cc.edu/~msheah/paper1.html/ on February 15, 2005.

Chapter Eight
Working Through Conflict

Taking charge of a patient care unit in a healthcare organization provides all the ingredients for conflict. As the charge nurse, you have the opportunity to prevent and manage conflicts. This is an exciting and challenging part of the job. Here's where you demonstrate your best interpersonal skills, your powers of negotiation and your intense focus on the patients.

There are different types of conflicts. The ability to recognize types of conflict is helpful in finding resolution. Is the conflict *internal* or *external*?

"A real leader faces the music even when he doesn't like the tune." — *Anonymous*

Internal Conflict

An *internal* conflict exists within you and is usually the easiest type to resolve. For example, you may feel the urge to lash out but, instead, you must smile and be polite. Getting beyond internal conflict requires self-control, self-awareness, maturity and choosing your battles. Sometimes you have to learn the hard way. Here's an example. I used to work with a physician who was very dramatic and verbal when it came to expressing her frustration. In my first few encounters with her, I kept trying to move the conversation beyond the phase of venting to the stage of communicating information, explanations and problem-solving. This, I learned, only prolonged the volume and length of the venting phase. I learned that my role was to listen attentively, not speak and wait patiently until the doctor had calmed down enough to converse. The conflict was really within me – it was *internal*. I had to learn how to prevent escalation of the situation by controlling my inner conflict. *Internal* conflicts usually involve strong feelings within you and require you to control your non-verbal behavior. Sighing, rolling the eyes or folding the arms defiantly across your chest will only prolong the conflict.

"Whenever you're in conflict with someone, there is one factor that can make the difference between damaging your relationship and deepening it. That factor is attitude."
— *Timothy Bentley, leadership author and coach*

External Conflict

External conflict is either *situational* or *interpersonal*.

- *Situational* conflicts are usually temporary and exist only in the moment. They often have to do with limited resources or incompatible priorities. For example, there is a last minute request for one of the nurses on your team to accompany her assigned patient to radiology. This request coincides with her designated lunch break. At the same time, a new admission (which has been pre-assigned to her) arrives on the unit. The conflict is that she needs to be in three places at once. She may be able to figure this out in collaboration with her teammates; however, it is very possible that she will come to you for help in reallocating the work load. At the very least, she needs your approval to shift the work — so that you always know who is taking care of whom, who is off the unit, etc. If *situational* conflicts are resolved quickly and objectively, they usually do not escalate. Make a decision based on data, announce the decision, explain your reasons and move forward. You really do not have time for negotiation or group process. Lead your team. People will be grateful if you resolve situational conflicts quickly and decisively.

"Whoever has the mind to fight has broken his connection with the universe. If you try to dominate people you are already defeated. We study how to resolve conflict, not how to start it."
— *Daniel Goleman, leadership author*

- The most difficult type of conflict to resolve is *interpersonal*. *Interpersonal* conflicts are often about something else, not the current issue. They may be about an ongoing struggle for power or control that exists between two people. Conflict may result when there are differing goals, ideas or interpretations of roles and priorities. The key is to recognize the conflict quickly and remain objective.

"In one's family, respect and listening are the source of harmony." — *Buddha, spiritual leader, 560-480 BC*

Be Alert to Potential Conflict

As a charge nurse, you get to know the people you work with and their character traits. After a while, you can predict who will become involved in conflicts and who will not. When you come on duty and are preparing for a shift, you learn to assess who is working with you and how they are feeling. Having a pulse and knowing which personalities are almost always a challenge helps you to be prepared.

What are the group dynamics? Is there light-heartedness and are people quietly and cooperatively going about their work? Or is there a feeling of sarcasm, anger, hostility and burn-out? Even worse, is there complete silence? Can you "cut the air with a knife?" Calling this to people's attention at shift report may help. "What's going on? Everyone seems distracted." Get it out; talk about it. Remind everyone to focus on the patients. Encourage everyone to work as a team. There are usually just one or two people who seem bent on everyone having a bad day. If it is necessary, pull these people aside and discuss the situation. Ask them for their help. If necessary, enlist the support of your supervisor and get beyond whatever is causing the problem. Set the tone and move on.

We all know people who thrive on conflict. They love to get everyone involved. Watch out for them! I used to have a supervisor who said, "When you see a freight train bearing down on you, get off the tracks or you will be crushed by it and become part of the problem. Let the train roll on by and hope that it will run out of steam when no one rushes to jump on. Keep an eye on this train, however, and if it gathers speed grab the brakes of conflict resolution."

"In dwelling, live close to the ground. In thinking, keep to the simple. In governing, don't try to control. In work, do what you enjoy. In family life, be completely present." — *Lao-Tzu, Chinese philosopher, 604 BC*

Coping Skills

People who are good at conflict prevention and management:

- see conflict as an opportunity for growth.
- read situations quickly.
- are good at active listening.
- can hammer out tough agreements and settle disputes equitably.
- can find common ground and get cooperation with minimal noise.
- focus on finding the *best* solution; not on winning or the people involved.
- focus on mutual respect and professionalism.
- instill an environment of working for a higher purpose: *what is best for the patient.*
- seek options and alternative strategies.
- instill trust and make decisions at the lowest level possible.

"Difficulties are meant to rouse, not discourage. The human spirit is to grow strong by conflict." — *William Ellery Channing, founder of Unitarianism*

If you find yourself faced with a conflict between two or more of the people upon whom you rely to be productive team members, you must act. Time spent in conflict and time spent in resolving it is time spent away from the patients. You do not have a lot of time to waste but even more time will be wasted if you do not act. Stepping up to the plate to resolve conflict takes courage, especially the first few times you have to do it. You gain confidence and skill each time. You gain respect. *Once people realize you will address conflict they will be less likely to engage in it.*

So, what do you do?

- Take a deep breath.
- Determine what you hope to accomplish.
- Remember that you are being observed and watched by everyone.
- Be professional and be a leader. Be kind, but unemotional.
- Think about the future and the positive effect of resolving the conflict.
- See the bigger picture. Step outside what is going on as if you could look at it from afar.
- Think win-win.
- Think of your role as a negotiator not as a combatant.
- Act quickly.
- Move participants in the conflict to a private area, if possible.
- Ask everyone to calm down.
- Downsize the conflict — ask everyone to remove the emotion and to stop the personal attacks.
- Ask participants to explain their points of view.
- Listen attentively and respectfully.
- Acknowledge the value of each point of view. Help everyone save face.
- Verbalize the common ground. "We all want Patient 'X' to…"
- State the nature of the conflict without personalizing it.
- Ask each participant to suggest a resolution.

- Bargain, trade and arbitrate.
- If participants cannot decide on a resolution, you must.
- State your decision, ask everyone to agree to it and then ask them to move on.
- If emotions and personal issues still remain, set a time when you will get together and discuss the issue at greater length — such as the end of the shift.
- Make sure that people follow through on the resolution that was reached or agreed upon.
- If necessary, keep your commitment to meet later. Include a third party, such as your supervisor, if everyone agrees this could help.

The step-by-step approach described above is an extreme move. You rarely need to go through all of these steps — people just don't have time for it and they come to their senses and realize they have to get beyond the conflict. Chances are you will reach a resolution much faster and with much greater ease than the above scenario suggests.

"The gem cannot be polished without friction, nor man perfected without trials." — *Confucius, Chinese philosopher, 551-479 BC*

A compounding factor is that one of the participants in a conflict may be a physician. All of the above suggestions still hold. There may be a perceived imbalance of power and possibly demeaning comments will be flung out in the heat of the conflict. Take charge. The patient's well-being is at risk. It has been my experience that if you act quickly, fairly and professionally to resolve the conflict, and if you do this consistently, the doctor will be appreciative of your intervention. Just as you know which doctors are most likely to become embroiled in non-productive spats, the doctors know which charge nurses are adept at getting the team back on track.

"Honest disagreement is often a sign of good progress." —
Gandhi, Indian leader

Be Prepared

As charge nurse you have to be prepared to handle conflict. It is an inevitable by-product of the intense human interaction that is the daily scene in a busy patient care unit. It is good in that it is the result of people really caring about what they do. Unfortunately, it can take the focus off the first priority — patient care.

Learning to handle conflict is one of the more demanding tasks that you must address as a charge nurse. It is stressful but, if you do it well, it can be exhilarating. It is hard to actually enjoy managing conflict but, if you find that you're good at it, you may want to consider a management position.

"A hero is no braver than an ordinary man, but he is brave five minutes longer." — *Ralph Waldo Emerson, author, poet, and philosopher*

Five Ways to Cope With Negative Colleagues
by Gary S. Topchik, *Managing Workplace Negativity*

People demonstrate their negative attitudes in many different ways. You can learn how to handle each one, but there are some general coping strategies.

Recognize that an attitude problem exists. The first step is to recognize that someone is expressing negativity in the workplace. Do not ignore it if it is affecting that person's performance, your performance, the performance of others or relationships with your clients or customers.

- Acknowledge any underlying causes for the negative attitude. As we know, negativity has many causes. The factors could include personal problems, work-related stress, a difficult boss, job insecurity, loss of loyalty, lack of growth or advancement opportunities and so forth. It helps to get the person to see the causes for his or her negativity. Ask non-threatening questions of colleagues like, "You look stressed. Can I help?" It is also important to recognize that what is causing the negativity is often justified and that the negativist has the right to feel that way.
- Help the person take responsibility. It is ultimately the responsibility of the negative person to change his or her negative attitude and behaviors at work. Even though the person may have every right to feel the way he or she does, it is still not appropriate for the workplace. As a team member or boss, you need to help your colleague recognize this and have him or her take ownership. Consider addressing the problem privately with the person in a way that demonstrates concern for both their problems and the well-being of the team.
- Replace negative, inappropriate reactions with different, more acceptable ones. Even though we just said that it is the job of a negativist to change his or her actions, you may need to help. The person may not know what to do differently to come across as more positive. It will often be up to you to specify exactly what that is. You can suggest that people aren't aware of the person's great qualities or that his contributions are being eclipsed by negative behavior.
- Instill positive attitudes in others. Be the role model for your negativists through your actions and behaviors. You can prevent their negativity by instilling in them the positivist bug. If you do that, they may never catch the negativity virus again.
- Most of all, it's important to start a dialogue with difficult colleagues so issues can be addressed.

Reprinted with permission

Case Study – Dennis

At County Medical when an RN "calls off," the others have to cover the shift to make ends meet. Dennis, RN, is a good technical nurse, but he is a complainer. He whines all the time, regardless of who is in earshot. A unit has had three nurses call off and Dennis is asked to "float" to that unit. Upon arrival at the other unit, Sandy (charge nurse) greets Dennis saying, "We're glad to have you as part of our team today. We like having people from other units help us."

Dennis answers, "This isn't what I was hired to do. I'm only here because I have to be." Sandy ignores this and explains how the unit operates; however, through the entire orientation, Dennis whines. This starts getting on Sandy's nerves, but she does not confront the behavior.

As the day goes on, others on the unit begin noticing Dennis' attitude, including one patient's family member who mentions it to a doctor who in turn tells Sandy. With so much going on, Sandy does not have (or take) time to deal with his behavior.

It is five hours into the shift, and Dennis has now offended three RNs. Sandy is at her limit. Two nurses have asked Sandy to take care of the issue. The unit is buzzing with drama, and the only one unaware of this is Dennis.

What is Sandy's next course of action? How does she resolve the conflict? How could all of this play out? After all, Sandy does not have any formal power over Dennis. What do you think?

Reflections

- How do I deal with conflict at work?
- What are my buttons or triggers? How do I respond when these buttons are pushed?

- Do I find myself getting involved in other people's conflict?
- Do I find myself avoiding conflict at all costs?
- I deal best with conflict when I...
- When others around me are in conflict, I feel...

Remember...

- Before you can help others through their conflicts, you need to be aware of how you deal with conflict. In other words, you need to be self-aware about your ways of working through conflict. Do you lash out? Withdraw? Avoid? Stay calm? You must first be in tune with yourself before you can lead others effectively.
- The most difficult type of conflict to resolve is *interpersonal. Interpersonal* conflicts are often about something else. They are often not about the current issue.
- *Situational* conflicts are usually temporary and exist only in the moment. *Situational* conflicts often have to do with limited resources or incompatible priorities.
- As charge nurse you have to be prepared to handle conflict. It is an inevitable by-product of the intense human interaction that is the daily scene in a busy patient care unit. It is good in that it is the result of people really caring about what they do. It is bad in that it takes the focus off of real work that must be done.

Additional Resources

- *The Eight Essential Steps to Conflict Resolution: Preserving Relationships at Work, at Home, and in the Community* by Dudley Weeks
- *Managing Disagreement Constructively: Conflict Management in Organizations* by Herbert S. Kindler
- *Managing Workplace Negativity* by Gary S. Topchik

- *Conflict Resolution* by Daniel Dana

References

Stewart, K. (2003). *A portable mentor for organizational leaders.* Portsmouth, Ohio: SOMCPress, Inc.

Topchik, G. (n.d.). Five Ways to Cope with Negative Colleagues. Retrieved from http://love.ivillage.com on December 13, 2004.

Chapter Nine
Patient Satisfaction & Service Recovery

"To provide appropriate service you have to know what your customer is feeling." — *Dan James, artist and author*

Until the early 1990s, not much thought was given to whether or not patients were satisfied. It was just assumed that they were doing okay, except for the occasional complainer. I remember the first time I heard that the hospital where I worked would conduct standardized, periodic surveys of our patients to assess their level of satisfaction. I was the director of nursing, and was assigned lead responsibility for analyzing the results. I was not worried. I was confident the patients would give us great ratings. Alas! They did not. The scores were all over the place.

Health care has been slower than other businesses — even other service industries — to study patient (customer) satisfaction. Looking back it is hard to understand why, since now it is standard operating procedure to do these surveys. Perhaps it was related to the fact that physicians and nurses strongly objected to the image of health care as a business and the identifying of patients as customers.

Several events, external to healthcare providers, took place in the last two decades of the 20th century that changed the way the healthcare industry behaved. The implementation of Diagnostic Related Groups (DRGs) decreased hospital revenue and caused healthcare organizations to look more carefully at where money comes from and where it goes. DRGs caused hospitals to shorten lengths of stay. This action resulted in dissatisfaction for both patients and physicians. To maintain a healthy bottom line, healthcare organizations needed to increase the number of patients served per year to fill the beds that were opened up as lengths of stay decreased.

During this same period of time, consumers became more educated and demanding. The old patriarchal system in which patients went wherever their doctors directed began to break down. Patients began to make choices whenever it was within their power to do so. Physicians became less loyal to any one healthcare organization. They took their patients to the healthcare organizations where they thought their patients were most satisfied. Additionally, mergers of healthcare systems began to take place, which broke down the old system of independent community healthcare organizations. Healthcare systems negotiated with third party payers for preferred provider status. Third party payers began to request information about clinical outcomes *and* patient satisfaction in an attempt to swing business to the providers where people would not only receive the best clinical care but also be most satisfied.

Health care became more competitive and businesslike. Although painful, these changes have been positive in that they have caused the quality of care to improve. The changes have caused us to do the right thing — improve patient satisfaction. We try harder now to treat patients in the way we would want to be treated. We are more aware of how we are perceived by patients.

"It is not the employer who pays the wages. Employers handle the money. It is the customer who pays the wages." — *Henry Ford, entrepreneur*

Lessons Learned

In recent years, much has been learned about patient satisfaction. There is enough cumulative data on this topic (nationwide) for the industry to draw some conclusions and implement improvements. We learned that meeting needs and exceeding patients' expectations is not easy. As healthcare organizations began to explore this topic, the experiences of other industries were studied. Existing databases and strategies on the topic of customer satisfaction were from industries very dissimilar to healthcare. Think about it. No one chooses to be in a hospital or nursing home.

The patients are virtual prisoners. We take their clothes, freedom of choice and dignity. They come to us not feeling well in the first place. Then, we poke and prod them, put them through unpleasant tests and procedures, and give them bad news ranging from tasteless diets to terminal diagnoses. Patients are anxious, frightened, angry and lonely.

We have learned that patient satisfaction is *not* a program. It is a change in philosophy. It is a change in the way we conduct ourselves each minute of the day. It works best when this change is systemic to the entire workplace. If we treat each other with dignity and respect, the entire culture becomes more caring and compassionate. Mutual respect is one of the most necessary ingredients in creating a healing environment — which, after all, is what nursing is all about.

We have also learned that in the minds of most patients, we are all responsible for each other's behaviors and actions. This means that patients really do not care who is to blame for what, they just want it fixed. If an inpatient has a bad time in the emergency department, the dissatisfaction experienced at the first point of contact can become a cloud of distrust and suspicion over the actions of all who care for the patient throughout the stay. If the discharge process does not go smoothly, this last moment of contact with the organization may cast a negative shadow over the memory of the entire experience. The goal of satisfaction is not one that can be achieved in the same sense that meeting the budget is achieved. An environment in which patients are consistently satisfied requires everyone's commitment and proactive performance all the time. It requires that everyone be "tuned in" to the individual needs of others.

"Be everywhere, do everything, and never fail to astonish the customer." — *Motto of Macy's, department store*

Drivers of Patient Satisfaction

The accumulated data tells us that there are a few factors that drive patient satisfaction. If these things happen for the patients, they are more likely to feel satisfied with their stay. These factors are more qualitative than quantitative; more subjective than objective. They are common sense and yet in the busy, sometimes impersonal world of healthcare organizations, they do not consistently occur. The two professional groups that are drivers of satisfaction are physicians and nurses (especially nurses). This is not surprising since these are the two groups of professionals the patients most associate with the healthcare organization. In the case of nurses, they are the group most frequently in contact with the patient.

Patients want people to introduce themselves by name, explain why they are in the room and what they are about to do. They want communication, information and education. They want to know what is going on with their tests and what will happen next. They want to know which doctor is doing what. They want to feel like partners in their own care and plan of treatment. They want clarification if they hear conflicting bits of information from different caregivers. Most of all, they want their nurses to be professional, warm, caring and compassionate.

"Perception is real even when it is not reality." — *Edward de Bono, leadership author*

Compounding Factors

Although this sounds easy enough, it is not. There are many reasons for this.

- Caregivers become so accustomed to the routine that they sometimes forget that it is all new and foreign to the patient, and that they need to take the time to explain everything — the environment, the daily schedule, who is doing what, etc.

- At times, nurses and other caregivers are so busy trying to do all things for all people that, to the patient, they don't appear to have the time to care or answer questions. It is a good habit to pause before you leave a patient's bedside, smile, take a breath and sincerely ask, "Is there anything else I can do for you? Do you have any questions? I have the time." Although you may think you don't have time, it will save you a lot of time in the long run. The mere act of asking these questions helps the patient relax and feel that you truly care.

- There are many people visiting the patients and, although patients may think we are communicating with one another, often we are not. Nurses can get blind-sided. A patient may ask, "Who was that doctor who just came to see me? I have never met her before. And why was she here? She told me something about a test she was ordering. Can you explain that to me? She was in such a hurry I felt as though she didn't have time for my questions." You may not know the answer. To the patient this is a simple question; to you it is not. There is so much going on it is not possible for you to know everything; however, patients see you — especially in the role of charge nurse — as all-knowing. Saying "I don't know" is the wrong response; however, if those words are quickly followed with "but I will find out and get right back to you," you are on the road to meeting the patient's needs.

- When other departments do something that is dissatisfying to a patient (e.g., bringing the wrong lunch tray or delaying an X-ray) the patient's frustration is often vented on the nurse. If you respond by saying, "That's not nursing's fault; that is radiology's fault," this only causes the patient to become more frustrated. Skip over whose fault it is. Thank the patient for letting you know of the problem and then proceed to fix it. Explain to the patient what you have done about the complaint.

- Sometimes the issue of improving patient satisfaction scores gets blown out of proportion. Administrators who do not take time to understand the complicated dynamics of patient care may focus only on the key drivers or the survey results. They think that, since the behavior and actions of nurses are so important in determining the patient's satisfaction level, it must be nursing's fault when the scores are lower than desired, which can result in an undeserved heavy-handedness toward nursing. In the worst case scenario, threats (or rumors of threats) may be made by management. You may hear something like, "If satisfaction scores don't improve, something bad is going to happen. People will be disciplined and fired." This, of course, creates a challenging environment. Nurses become afraid to do what is best for the patient because it may cause the patient to become dissatisfied. For example, a doctor orders a patient to get out of bed and sit in a chair for a couple of hours each shift. If the patient doesn't feel like getting out of bed and sitting up, the nurse may let the patient stay in bed out of fear of dissatisfying the patient. This is not good. If you see this happening, you need to talk about it in a staff meeting or with your supervisor. Get it out on the table. You can't let bad management get in the way of good nursing care.

"Organizations have more to fear from lack of internal customer service than from any level of external customer service." — *Ron Tillotson, performance improvement author*

- There are a few people who do not seem to want to be satisfied. This is true inside and outside of healthcare organizations. Their cups are half empty. The best approach is for you and your team to develop a nursing plan of care that emphasizes a consistent approach.
- On the flip side, there is a percentage of patients who are always sweet, pleasant, optimistic and forgiving. Their cups are more than half full. Only the very worst events will cause them to be dissatisfied. They make up another five percent or so of the patient mix. It is the 90 percent in the middle who need that extra caring and communication to feel satisfied. It is this same 90 percent who give the most honest and helpful feedback in surveys.

- The ideal approach to satisfying patients is to *do it right the first time*. As legendary basketball coach John Wooden once said, "If you don't have the time to do it right the first time, when will you have the time to do it over?"

If patients feel satisfied and secure in the care they receive, they will likely be positive and accepting of every interaction; however, this does not happen often. Consequently, nurses are placed in the position of *service recovery* — trying to turn a negative or frustrating experience into a positive one. This takes more effort and consistency. The playing field is not level. The patient may be anxious, watchful, fearful, doubtful, pessimistic and not as trusting as if all had gone well from the start.

As charge nurse, your role in patient satisfaction can be more demanding and complex than the clinical aspects of the position. However, your *patient satisfaction* role can be detailed in the following manner:

- meet the needs of every patient you encounter.
- meet the needs of every person giving care or service to you or your team of nurses.
- act as a role model at all times.
- assess the level of every patient as you do rounds and follow-up if needed — this includes praising the staff and alerting it of potential issues.
- ask every patient if there is something more you can do for him or her.
- perform the miracles of service recovery.

"Reality doesn't bite, rather our perception of reality bites."
— *Anthony D'Angelo, leadership author*

Service Recovery

As charge nurse you will most likely get involved in service recovery when a patient is upset. He or she has probably just said to the direct care giver, "I want to speak to your supervisor." If you are lucky, there is one more chance to turn things around before the patient picks up the phone to let someone in administration know about the terrible service.

"Good judgment comes from experience. And where does experience come from? Experience comes from bad judgment."
— *Mark Twain, author*

Many nurses are very good at service recovery. Some are not so good, and become frustrated and defensive. Here are some helpful steps for service recovery situations.

- Respond promptly, if possible. If not, send a message to the patient or tell them in person that you will be able to come in "X" minutes. Clarify expectations for the patient. Bear in mind that any amount of waiting makes the problem worse. Therefore, it is a good idea to give a brief reason for any unavoidable delay. For example you could say, "I must return a physician's call before I am available. That will take about 10 minutes and then I will come to talk with you." Then do as you have promised and return to the patient in 10 minutes or less.
- Act in a calm, courteous and professional manner. Address the patient as "Ms." or "Mr."
- Apologize. Say "I am sorry that you are unhappy." This is a powerful statement. It acknowledges that the patient is not satisfied and that you will try to fix the problem. It does not mean you are guilty or at fault.
- Trust the patient. Listen actively and attentively. Clarify. Ask questions. Repeat the story so that you and the patient are on the same wave length. Try to understand not only the facts, but also the patient's feelings. Make an

empathetic statement such as, "I can see why you are frustrated." Be open. Do not be defensive. Do not talk about who is at fault. Be aware of your non-verbal communication, which can sometimes aggravate patients.

- Take on the problem. Explain that you will investigate and attempt to fix the problem and then come back and tell the patient what you have done to correct the issue.
- Act quickly. If you do not have time to investigate immediately and resolve the issue, delegate it to someone who is reliable, accurate and quick.
- Follow-up with the patient. Explain what you have done to fix the problem. If possible, explain that it is fixed in such a way that it will not happen to another patient. This places the patient in the role of hero and erases any guilt he may feel for complaining.
- If there is a barrier to fixing the issue, admit it. "I'm sorry, but radiology cannot do your test today because of several emergency patients. It will be done tomorrow." Then ask, "Is there anything else that you need or that I can do for you?" Be careful with this question because, if you insert it at the wrong time or say it in the wrong way, it can make the situation worse. It may sound as though you are talking down. Use your judgment. Follow the Golden Rule.
- Check with the patient a few hours later or the next day. Convey your sincere apology again and communicate the message that you want the patient to have the best possible experience. Help the patient see you as an advocate.

Patient Satisfaction Feedback

As a nurse you should learn as much as you can about the patient satisfaction process in your healthcare organization. What survey is used? What questions are asked? What are the trends in scores? What happens to unsolicited feedback? Is this compiled and trended? What do these trends show? What are the drivers that indicate repeat business or referred business for your healthcare organization? Are results available specifically for your department or unit? What is being done well? What initiatives have been implemented to improve scores — such as suggested scripts to help people say the right things at the right times? Can you get on a committee or task force to help with these initiatives?

From a positive perspective, a complaint can be thought of as a gift. Patients see things from a perspective that is fresh and different. When they verbalize complaints or feedback, patients are often providing valuable feedback. Addressing concerns allows patients to feel valued, relaxed and, therefore, better prepared to heal. Think of complaints as gifts. Thinking of them as irritants gets you nowhere.

"Customer complaints are the schoolbook from which we learn." — *Anonymous*

Terms & Acronyms

- **DRGs** — Diagnosis Related Groups. A patient classification system that provides a way to describe types of patients. DRGs are the basis of the system used by Medicare to pay healthcare providers.

Forbidden Phrases

The following **forbidden phrases** tend to inflame situations. What **acceptable phrase** could be used in its place?

Forbidden Phrase	Correct Phrase
"You'll have to…"	
"I'll have to…"	
"I don't know."	

Forbidden Phrase	Correct Phrase

"We can't do that."

"You misunderstood me."

"We are short staffed."

"Hang on a second, I'll be back."

Case Study – An Unforgettable Flight

Imagine you have never flown in an airplane, but tomorrow morning you will have to take your first flight with your five-year-old son across the country. Much to your dismay the flight will take five hours, so you will have to wake up at least three hours before that. You are nervous because you have never flown before. You are afraid of flying. You are nervous for your child's safety as well as your own. Images of that horrible story on the news race through your mind along with every movie that ever had a bad scene about airplanes. For some reason, that's all you can think about. Those with whom you have spoken brush off your fears and say, "It's safe. You'll be fine!"

The morning of the flight, there is a huge thunderstorm coming through the area, which does not help things. Bravely, you make your way to the airport and prepare for your flight. After waiting 30 minutes in line, the first person you encounter is the baggage agent. She appears stressed out and is curt with you. She checks your bags and says, "Gate 17C, over there." Having never been in the airport, "over there" was not much help. Before you can ask a follow-up question, the man behind you is already checking in.

You wander around and find a sign for Terminal C. You move through security where they make you take off your shoes and pull you aside to search your carry-on luggage. They not only go through your things, but also frisk you and ask you to take off your belt, etc. You ask why they are doing this and the agent responds,

"It's policy. They make us do this, ever since 9/11." Your child starts crying. Your anxiety level rises.

Finally, you arrive at your gate. Your flight is delayed. You wait in line for 15 minutes and ask the gate agent how long the delay will be. She looks at you and says, "It could be up to two hours. Can I do anything for you?" You respond, "No" and sit down. The gate area is packed with people. Children are crying and your son is becoming restless. Two hours turn into three. You look outside and notice that the storm has not subsided — in fact, the weather looks worse.

At last, it is time to go. The agent mentions that some work needed to be done on the plane. Thoughts run through your head. What does this mean? Are we going to crash? Is this plane not in good shape? You want to call your husband but, by this time, you are being herded onto the plane. As you pass the cockpit, you see all kinds of buttons, lights and knobs. The pilots are working frantically and, as you are looking, the flight attendant interrupts and asks you to move along to your seat.

You sit down and place all of your attention on taking care of your son. Because of this, you miss all the pre-flight instructions. A flight attendant comes by and snaps, "Ma'am put your tray table up and stow that bag. You are holding us up!" At this point, you want to cry. You look out the window at gray skies and rain. The engines begin. You hear strange noises. Finally, you are in the air. The majority of the flight is filled with turbulence. At one point, even the flight attendants have to sit down.

At long last, you land and as you are leaving the plane, the flight attendant says, "Hope you had a great flight! Come fly with us again!"

You can see where this is going. The majority of patients you see every day are flying for the first time. For them, everything is stormy. They are worried about their children; they are worried about their safety. They do not understand the machines in the room. They do not understand clinical language and they do not understand what is happening to their bodies. All they know is that they are on a flight they never wanted to take; however, they do know one thing — they know how they *feel*. It is really the only thing they can count on at this point. All other power has been taken away.

If they do not *feel* good, if things in the environment are aggravating them, if they do not understand, if they have had to wait a long time or if they perceive a negative attitude from an employee, you know the results. It is likely that as charge nurse, you will encounter these people "on a bad flight." Try to put yourself in their shoes, and try to view the situation from their point of view. This will help you empathize and work through their issues. Often they just want to vent and know that you care. Finally, remember that family members are on the flight as well. They are also along for an unpleasant ride and, understandably, they are not at their best either.

Review questions:

- How does the story parallel health care?
- What are the aggravators in healthcare organizations?
- Which factors can we manage and improve?
- How can scripting help prevent bad flights?
- How can patient education help prevent bad flights?
- How do you react when people around you are on bad flights? Anger? Frustration? What puts *you* on a bad flight?
- What can be done to turn bad flights into good ones?

Reflections

- Has there been a time recently when you received poor customer service? Where were you? What problems did you experience?
- How did those serving you respond to your complaints or concerns? Was there a sincere apology or did it feel forced?

- Were the problems you encountered systems problems (flawed processes) or were they personality problems?
- What are the most frequent complaints on your unit?
- Are the complaints due to personalities or broken systems? What service recovery training have individuals received on your unit?

Remember...

- We have learned that patient satisfaction is <u>not</u> a program. It is a change in philosophy. It is a change in the way we conduct ourselves each minute of the day. It works best when this change is systemic.
- The goal of satisfaction is not one that can ever be achieved in the sense that meeting the budget is achieved. An environment in which patients are consistently satisfied requires everyone's commitment all the time.
- Patients want people to introduce themselves by name, explain why they are in the room and what they are about to do. They want communication, information and education.
- As charge nurse, your role in patient satisfaction can be more demanding and complex than the clinical aspects of the position.
- As a nurse you should learn as much as you can about the patient satisfaction process used in your healthcare organization. What survey is used? What are the trends in scores? What happens to unsolicited feedback? Is this compiled and trended?
- Pay close attention to the perceptions of the patients with whom you are working. The more you can see things through their eyes, the more attentive you will be to their needs.

Additional Service Recovery Resources

- *Knock Your Socks Off Service Recovery* by Ron Zemke & Chip R. Bell
- *Resolving Patient Complaints*: *A Step-By-Step Guide to Effective Service Recovery* by Liz A. Osborne
- *If Disney Ran Your Hospital, 9 1/2 Things You Would Do Differently* by Fred Lee
- Video: *It's a Dog's World*

Chapter Ten
Patient Safety & Error Prevention

"Nursing is above all a provocative calling. Year by year, nurses have to learn new and improved methods. Year by year, nurses are called upon to do more and better than they have ever done." — *Florence Nightengale*

"Are the patients safe? Of course they are. Patient safety is *job No.1*. What are you talking about? Your data is wrong. Patient safety is the basis of everything we do. The concept of patient safety is intrinsic to every one of our practices and procedures."

These were my thoughts when I first heard about the Institute of Medicine's (IOM) 1999 report entitled *To Err is Human: Building a Safer Health System*. This report stated that between 44,000 and 98,000 people in the United States die annually because of errors in patient care. This report caught the attention of the media, the public, third party payers and healthcare providers. It was much quoted and discussed. It resulted in further studies and reports. The most important thing about these reports and studies is that they have inspired the healthcare industry to look more objectively at its practices and outcomes. It has caused us to make changes in the way health care is provided and the quality indicators we monitor.

After my initial thoughts of denial and disbelief, I became more rational and objective. In fact, I began to realize that there has been a sort of "conspiracy of silence" about errors and "near misses" that happen or almost happen to patients. I thought back to a scene that took place when I was a student nurse. In my initial surgical rotation, I scrubbed in on a case as an observer. During intubation the patient's front tooth was dislodged. A voice at the table said, "No one saw this happen." I was shocked. It was the first time I had witnessed the harming of a patient. It was an accident. It was not intentional. But the fact that a "cover-up" was the first verbalized plan to handle this harm to a patient was unconscionable to me. I discussed it with my nursing instructor.

She assured me it was only a casual remark, maybe even an attempt at humor. But I thought about it a lot and have never forgotten it. Nor have I forgotten the way I felt about it.

Every nurse has had some encounter with the wrong side of patient safety. We have found errors made by others, found a "near miss" or even made an error ourselves. Chances are that if you have made an error you will never forget it. Many errors are probably never discovered; however, making a mistake leaves a lasting memory of how easily it can happen. It makes you a believer in reform. Any change in process or procedure that will prevent errors and harm to the patients is definitely a good idea.

Errors happen and patient safety is vulnerable because our systems and processes are not as error-proof as they should and can be. People are blamed and punished and feel at fault, but it is the steps we go through, the complexity of our systems, the many hands a dangerous medication passes through before it gets to the patient that need to be the focus of our scrutiny and reform. Can we make things simpler, more foolproof and secure? How can we change the system to prevent an error in the future? These are the questions we must constantly ask ourselves. Continuous improvement does not result from thinking in terms of fault or who is to blame for an error. Continuous improvement comes from studying every error and "near miss" to better understand how the process or system can be changed to prevent or decrease the likelihood of errors in the future. Continuous improvement will happen more quickly if people feel that reporting an error is a good thing. It will lead to greater safety for patients. It is a barrier to safety if people feel that reporting an error will get them or another person "in trouble." We are making progress in creating blame-free environments and increasing patient safety; but we have a long way to go. In fact, this journey will never end.

"It may seem strange to enunciate as the very first requirement in a hospital that it should do the sick no harm." — *Florence Nightengale*

Patient Safety is a Priority

You are responsible for many things as a charge nurse. The most important of these is the safety of the patients. Your top priority is patient safety. You have to help everyone remember it is their priority too. You are the patient's advocate in this as in all things. Clarity in communication is the best way to meet this challenge. Special care must be taken when receiving telephone and verbal orders. Repeating what you have heard is an excellent way to clarify that the sender and receiver agree upon what has been said. Be precise about what you are delegating and what you expect to be done. Act aggressively to intervene when a patient's condition deteriorates. Make assignments based upon patient safety. Resolving conflicts and calming emotions are important factors in the prevention of errors. A survey of physicians and nurses was conducted in 50 Veterans Health Administration hospitals with 1,500 participants. The majority of respondents stated that they believe disruptive behavior causes adverse events and medical errors, and has an adverse effect on patient safety, patient mortality, quality of care and patient satisfaction.

It is unfortunate, but likely, that sometimes you will have the responsibility for following up when an error has been made. Be proactive. Ask your supervisor what steps you should follow. Do your best to avoid a blaming environment. Focus on the process that went wrong and not on the people involved. One of the ways we can continuously improve care is to create an environment of acceptance and forgiveness instead of one of blame and fear. When an error is made and reported, it is an opportunity to investigate the root cause(s) and then change the systems or processes that have allowed an unsafe act to occur. This is a cultural change, but it *must* happen if we are to reach our goal of zero tolerance for errors.

Much has happened since the IOM report in 1999 and a lot more will happen. Mandates are constantly coming down regarding patient safety. External regulatory agencies and third party payers are all demanding changes. Good suggestions are coming to us from within and outside the healthcare industry. Many are being implemented. The adaptation of electronic information systems will help resolve the issues of illegible handwriting, transcription errors and incompatible orders, *but it still comes down to the person-to-person interaction that is the essence of health care.* No amount of changes in systems will substitute for each person taking personal responsibility for what they do or do not do for the patient.

"The safety of the people is the supreme law." — *Cicero, Roman philosopher, 106-43 BC*

Health Care is Becoming Safer

Some of what must be done is beyond the control of an individual nurse, but it is good to be aware of what is happening. It helps to know how intensely healthcare is being scrutinized and how seriously we must take the issue of patient safety. It also helps to know that we are surrounded by efforts designed to make our practice safer.

Soon after the IOM report, a group of *Fortune 500* executives external to health care formed the Leapfrog Group. Their organizations are the largest purchasers of healthcare coverage. Their interest stemmed not only from their concern that their employees were receiving safe care, but also from their concern regarding the exorbitant cost of health care. Every error costs money. They wanted to know that good dollars were not being wasted on bad medicine. The Leapfrog Group studied the hospital environment. Businesses external to health care are much more advanced in safety programs, which is sad, but true. As objective observers — skilled at designing safe environments — they made some suggestions. These are three changes they believe will decrease errors and improve patient outcomes:

1. Implementation of Computerized Physician Order Entry (CPOE).
2. Critical care units staffed with physicians trained as intensivists.
3. Evidence-based hospital referral for high risk procedures. Patients should be directed to healthcare organizations for

high risk surgeries and procedures based upon the number of similar procedures done by that healthcare organization, as well as the history of outcomes. In other words, complex procedures should be done in places where there is evidence that a large number of these procedures have been done safely and with success.

These concepts make a lot of sense. Many healthcare organizations are in the process of implementing them; however, there are barriers that may impede rapid, wide-scale adaptation of these changes. The barriers are expense, the physician reimbursement system, traditional referral patterns and the trend toward every community healthcare organization offering nearly every procedure. These changes will take time and money, and are easier said than done. Some of these changes reach beyond the ability of individual healthcare organizations to fix. They require changes in the "bigger system."

"You wouldn't just decide to forget about recovering the black box after an air crash. So why should it be thought so strange to learn from every accident in healthcare?" — *Sir Liam Donaldson, British physician and author*

JCAHO and Safety

The Joint Commission for the Accreditation of Healthcare Organizations (JCAHO) has always had patient safety embedded in its criteria. We have become accustomed to changes in the criteria that reflect that agenda. Beginning in 2004, JCAHO implemented *National Patient Safety Goals*, which are excellent goals. Healthcare organizations are monitored for compliance to these goals, and accreditation hinges upon implementation. As time goes on and as technology and techniques change there will be additions and refinements to JCAHO's patient safety goals. The seven goals implemented in 2004 were:

1. **Improve the accuracy of patient identification.** There will be two points of identification used for each patient

and neither of these may be the patient's room number. There will be a moment of final verification prior to surgery or any invasive procedure.

2. **Improve the effectiveness of communication among caregivers.** There will be verification/read back for telephone and verbal orders and for test results. There will be standardization of abbreviations, acronyms and symbols.

3. **Improve the safety of using high-alert medications.** Concentrated electrolytes will be removed from patient care units. There will be standardization and a limit in the number of drug concentrations on hand.

4. **Eliminate wrong-site, wrong-patient, wrong-procedure surgery.** There will be a pre-operative verification or checklist. The surgical site will be marked and, if possible, the patient will do this.

5. **Improve the safety of using infusion pumps.** Pumps must be designed to prevent free-flow infusion.

6. **Improve the effectiveness of clinical alarm systems.** There will be a schedule of regular preventative maintenance and testing that is adhered to. Alarms will be activated, will have appropriate settings and will be audible.

7. **Reduce the risk of healthcare acquired infections.** There will be compliance to the Centers for Disease Control and Prevention (CDC) hand hygiene guidelines. The institution will handle as Sentinel Events any deaths or losses of function that result from care or lack of care.

Every year the JCAHO National Patient Safety Goals are refined and expanded. Visit www.jcaho.org for the latest updates.

"The healthcare system, as it is currently structured, cannot consistently deliver effective care in a safe, timely and efficient manner." — *Institute of Medicine*

Become familiar with the work of the Institute for Healthcare Improvement (IHI), headed by Donald Berwick, M.D. This is an organization that has been working for many years through multidisciplinary collaboratives to improve the way we deliver care to patients. Visit their web site at www.ihi.org. They do exciting and hopeful work through real caregivers working in real healthcare settings. In December 2004, IHI launched a campaign to save 100,000 lives in U.S. healthcare organizations by June 14, 2006. It is called the "100K Lives Campaign." The plan is for participating healthcare organizations to implement the following six quality improvement changes.

1. **Deploy Rapid Response Teams** by allowing any staff member, regardless of position in the chain of command, to call upon a specialty team to examine a patient at the first sign of decline.

2. **Deliver Reliable Evidence-Based Care for Acute Myocardial Infarction** by consistently delivering key measures — including early administration of aspirin and beta-blockers — that prevent patient deaths from heart attack.

3. **Prevent Adverse Drug Events** by implementing medication reconciliation, which requires that a list of all of a patient's medications (even for unrelated illnesses) be compiled and reconciled to ensure that the patient is given (or prescribed) the right medications at the correct dosages — at admission, discharge and upon transfer of a patient to another care unit.

4. **Prevent Central Line Infection** by consistently delivering five interdependent, scientifically-grounded steps collectively called the "Central Line Bundle."

5. **Prevent Surgical Site Infections** by reliably delivering the correct perioperative antibiotics, maintaining glucose levels and avoiding shaving hair at the surgical site.

6. **Prevent Ventilator-Associated Pneumonia** by implementing five interdependent, scientifically-grounded steps, such as elevating the head of the bed by 30 degrees,

thereby dramatically reducing mortality and length of stay in the Intensive Care Unit.

"It is better to be safe than sorry." — *American proverb*

Nursing Care and Patient Safety

It is generally agreed by all who study patient safety that nurses as individuals, and as a professional group, are amenable to changes that will benefit patients. In fact, there is evidence that nurses are more able to see and to admit that change is needed. Perhaps this is because nurses are at the bedside and see errors and the negative consequences to patients.

In any case, the nursing profession has become more astute and proactive at monitoring patient outcomes that are the direct result of nursing interventions (or the lack thereof). Nurses identify and define key indicators, monitor patient outcomes and from the results, create *databases of nursing actions* that have a direct effect on the well-being of patients. Some examples are:

- Pressure ulcers
- Patient falls
- Restraint usage
- Aspiration pneumonia
- Medication errors
- Malnutrition
- Failure to follow physician orders
- Failure to have patients cough, deep breathe and ambulate
- Correlation of outcomes to staffing plans, skill mix, acuity, ADT and productivity

There is a growing body of knowledge known as Evidence-Based Nursing (EBN) or Evidence-Based Practice (EBP), which defines and hastens the process of embedding the findings of nursing research into clinical practice. It advocates the integration of the conscientious use of *best evidence* in combination with a *clinician's expertise* as well as *patient preferences and values* to make decisions about the care provided to patients.

Traditionally, it has taken as long as 15-20 years for evidence from nursing research to translate into clinical practice, which means care has been given that is not the safest for the patient even when there is evidence or proof of a better way. For example, nurses continued to change intravenous dressings daily long after there was significant evidence that this *increased* the rate of infection. To provide safer patient care we need to shorten this gap between scientific evidence and clinical practice. EBP is pioneering the way to do this. Enter "Evidence-Based Practice" into your internet search engine to learn more.

"I just try to be the best I can be and hope that is the best ever."
— *Tiger Woods, golfer*

Performance Improvement and You

It is likely that you are involved in performance improvement initiatives. If you are not, get involved because you can make a difference for the patients, your colleagues and yourself. Find out what indicators are being monitored for your nursing unit and how often. Find out how the data is collected. Ask about the results, trends, goals and to what the results are compared. Are the results compared to any external benchmarks or best practices? What is being done to improve results? What is the trigger that signals the need to do a root cause analysis? What is a root cause analysis? Is investigation being done to find out how similar nursing units are getting better results for the same indicators? Are the excellent results from your nursing unit being communicated to the rest of the healthcare organization? How? Is someone writing an article for a nursing journal to communicate this good news and these excellent practices to the rest of the nursing world? No? Then you could do that!

"Pleasure in the job puts perfection in the work."
— *Aristotle, Greek philosopher, 384-322 BC*

Safety through Communication

One final thought — be aware of the need to communicate with the patient in an understandable manner. This is essential for patient safety. Is the patient too anxious to listen? Can the patient hear? Can the patient see? Can the patient read? Can the patient understand and comprehend? Are you taking the time to listen to the patient? Does the patient have a failing memory? What language does the patient use? How do you get an interpreter? Use words from the patient's vocabulary, not the medical vocabulary. Interpret what the doctor said if the patient does not understand the message. For example, "The doctor said my test was positive. Is that good or is that bad?" All of this is simple and basic. You, of course, know this inside and out. It bears reflecting upon in the light of patient safety.

"The operation of a healthcare service depends upon a complex interaction between the patient, the environment in which care is provided and the people, equipment and facilities that deliver the care." — *Sir Liam Donaldson, British physician and author*

Terms & Acronyms

- **Acuity** — A term used to describe the severity of illness of patients, nurse dependency, complexity of care and similar factors used in the determination of staffing plans.
- **Average Length of Stay (ALOS)** — Refers to the average length of time that a patient stays in a nursing unit, hospital or extended care facility.
- **Admission, Transfer, Discharge (ATD)** — measures of the activity level of a patient care department.
- **Benchmark** — A goal to be attained or a "stretch" goal. These goals are used to compare results with other

providers. They can be found by consulting statistical reports available or are drawn from the best practices within the organization or industry. Benchmarks are used in quality improvement programs to encourage the improvement of care.

- **Centers for Disease Control & Prevention (CDC)** — "The Centers for Disease Control and Prevention (CDC) is recognized as the lead federal agency for protecting the health and safety of people — at home and abroad, providing credible information to enhance health decisions, and promoting health through strong partnerships. CDC serves as the national focus for developing and applying disease prevention and control, environmental health, and health promotion and education activities designed to improve the health of the people of the United States" (www.cdc.gov).
- **CMS** — Center for Medicare and Medicaid Services.
- **CPOE** — Computerized physician order entry.
- **HPPD or RVUs** — Hours Per Patient Day or Relative Value Units. Terms of measurement used to calculate staffing plans, budgets and productivity.
- **Length of Stay (LOS)** — the number of hours or days that a patient stays in a nursing unit or healthcare facility.
- **Root Cause Analysis** — A process used to find the underlying real cause(s) of a problem.
- **Sentinel Event** — An unexpected occurrence involving death, serious physical or psychological injury, or the risk thereof. Serious injury specifically includes loss of limb or function. Sentinel events signal the need for root cause analysis and correction.
- **Staffing Plan** — A plan that prescribes the allocation of human resources needed to care for a set of patients given certain conditions. For example, the skill mix and nurse-patient ratio needed on the 11-7 shift for a medical-surgical unit of an acute care hospital. This plan serves not only to determine staffing needs, but also budgetary needs. It includes both direct and indirect care.
- **Third party payers** — Entities or organizations that are primarily responsible to pay for medical care provided,

(e.g., health care insurers, CMS, worker's compensation programs, etc.) based upon contractual agreements.

Patient Safety in the News

Overworking Nurses has Adverse Effects on Patient Safety

July 9, 2004

A nationwide study co-authored by a Grand Valley State University nursing professor found that the long hours worked by hospital staff nurses may have adverse effects on patient safety.

Dr. Linda Scott, Grand Valley associate professor of nursing in the Kirkhof College of Nursing, said after studying the work habits of 393 hospital staff nurses, the research team found that nurses working more than 12.5 consecutive hours were three times more likely to make an error than nurses working shorter hours. Working overtime at the end of a shift also increased the risk of making an error.

The study, led by University of Pennsylvania nursing professor Dr. Ann Rogers will be published in the Journal of Health Affairs [July/August 2004]. The study was conducted by giving nurses logbooks to track hours worked, overtime, days off and sleep/wake patterns for 28 days. Participants were asked to describe errors or near errors that might have occurred during their work periods.

Participants reported 199 errors and 213 near errors during the data-gathering period. More than half the errors (58 %) involved medication administration; other errors included procedural errors (18 %), charting errors (12 %), and transcription errors (7 %).

Researchers found that most hospital nurses no longer work eight-hour day, evening or night shifts. Instead, they may be scheduled for 12-hour, 16-hour or even 20-hour shifts. Even when working extended shifts (over 12.5 hours), they were rarely able to leave the hospital at the end of their scheduled shift. All participants reported working overtime at least once during the data-gathering period and one-third of the nurses reported working overtime every day they worked.

"Both the use of extended shifts (over 12 hours) and overtime documented in this study pose significant threats to patient safety," Rogers said. "In fact, the routine use of 12-hour shifts should be curtailed and overtime – especially overtime associated with 12-hour shifts – should be eliminated."

The study was funded with a grant from the Agency for Healthcare Research and Quality in Maryland. Scott and Rogers are conducting a correlating study to research the work hours of critical care nurses.

Scott and Rogers are expected to speak before their respective state legislatures on nurse fatigue and patient safety. Scott is also working with the Michigan Nurses Association on patient safety legislation.

"We need to educate nurses and hospitals about fatigue," she said. "It's a shared responsibility and both parties are accountable. This is a national problem and will likely have a national effect."

Reprinted with permission

Patient Safety Quick Facts

According to the Institute of Medicine:

- In 1999, the Institute of Medicine released a report entitled *To Err is Human: Building a Safer Health System*. The report estimated that approximately 98,000 patients die *each year* as a result of healthcare errors in hospitals. This is more than the number of annual deaths from motor vehicle accidents, breast cancer or AIDS.

- From 1983 to 1993 there was a 250 percent increase in the number of deaths caused by medication errors.
- As of 2003, JCAHO reported that the number of Sentinel Events (unexpected deaths and serious injuries) reported each year continues to rise.

JCAHO & National Patient Safety Goals

"The purpose of the Joint Commission's National Patient Safety Goals is to promote specific improvements in patient safety. The goals highlight problematic areas in health care and describe evidence and expert-based solutions to these problems. Recognizing that sound system design is intrinsic to the delivery of safe, high quality health care, the goals focus on system-wide solutions, wherever possible" (www.jcaho.org).

Each year a new set of National Patient Safety Goals are set forth and, as care givers, you and your team should be aware of them.

These goals are developed based upon the Joint Commission's safety newsletter *Sentinel Event Alert*. According to JCAHO, "The Sentinel Event database, which contains de-identified aggregate information on sentinel events reported to the Joint Commission, is the primary, but not the sole, source of information from which the Alerts, as well as the National Patient Safety Goals, are derived" (www.jcaho.org).

Case Study – Rhonda

One day when you are in charge, Rhonda (an RN member of your team) approaches you and says, "I have called Dr. X to tell him that Mrs. Y is having chest pains. He is rounding in the CCU right now and will be here in a few minutes." You note that the doctor arrives on your unit and goes promptly to the room of Mrs. Y. He comes out of her room and states that he wants Mrs. Y transferred to CCU right away. He enters some notes and orders on her chart and then leaves. You call CCU to arrange for a bed. You then inform Rhonda of the doctor's visit and his order to transfer Mrs. Y to CCU ASAP. You tell her that CCU is ready for the transfer and that she is responsible for calling report and transferring the patient, and for checking Mrs. Y's chart for other pending orders. Rhonda says, "OK."

Ten minutes go by and you are aware that Mrs. Y has not been transferred to CCU. You find Rhonda in another patient's room and she says she can not do the transfer right away. You ask Jane, who is sitting at the nurses station working on the computer, if she could transfer the patient. She tells you she is busy doing some charting. You see Sue and Ellen standing in a corner talking. You ask if either of them could transfer Mrs. Y. They both say she is not their patient. You see two physicians at the desk who are asking to speak with you, but you decide you must leave your charge duties and transfer Mrs. Y yourself.

After you have completed the transfer you find Rhonda and tell her you have taken care of everything. Rhonda says, "I was going to do that in a minute. I didn't think it was that urgent." You say, "Oh, that's okay. I just wanted you to know that Mrs. Y is now in CCU."

You return to the desk to find that Jane is still at the computer. Sue and Ellen are still talking in the corner and there are several STAT orders that have not been taken care of. The unit secretary says that the doctors who had wanted to talk with you earlier want you to call their offices right away to talk about why their orders never get followed correctly on this unit.

- How does this story relate to patient safety?
- How did you miss out on providing good care in this situation? What could be done next time?
- What expectations must be set for your team?
- How will you help your team understand the importance of the situation?
- What are five things you must do to improve communication on your unit?

- What are five ways to provide feedback to your team members with performance issues?
- What resources/tools may assist you in this situation?

Reflections

- What processes on your unit lend themselves to errors?
- How many of these can be fixed with relative ease?
- Would those in positions of authority have any clue that these systems are broken and need fixing? If not, how could you communicate these safety issues?
- What is your role in patient safety and error prevention? Does it have a large effect on the organization?
- How can organizations such as JCAHO or the National Patient Safety Foundation help you in your job?

Remember...

- Patient safety is job No.1 for you as charge nurse. It is *the* most important thing that nurses do.
- When systems and processes do not lend themselves to safe practice or have high potential for error, it is your responsibility to let someone know. Perhaps it is your supervisor or someone in the quality department.
- There are a number of resources at your fingertips. Utilize them and stay knowledgeable about current trends and issues.

Additional Resources

- *National Patient Safety Foundation* (NPSF) — The Mission of the NPSF is "To Improve the Safety of Patients through our efforts to: Identify and create a core body of knowledge; Identify pathways to apply the knowledge; Develop and enhance the culture of receptivity to patient safety; Raise public awareness and foster communications about patient safety, and Improve the status of the Foundation and its ability to meet its goals" (www.npsf.org).

- *Joint Commission on Accreditation of Healthcare Organizations (JCAHO)* — The Mission of JCAHO is "To continuously improve the safety and quality of care provided to the public through the provision of healthcare accreditation and related services that support performance improvement in healthcare organizations" (www.jcaho.org).

- *Patient Safety Institute* — "Patient Safety Institute (PSI) is the healthcare industry's response to the need for a trusted, National Medical Information Exchange (NMIE) that provides real time access to critical patient information (with patient consent) at the point of care" (www.ptsafety.org).

- *The Bergendahl Institute* — "The Bergendahl Institute was established to transfer to the Healthcare Industry, 25 years of proven human error management techniques from the U.S. Nuclear Power Industry. The Institute's mission is to reduce medical errors, improve patient safety programs and strengthen safety cultures" (www.bergendahlinstitute.com).

- *HealthGrades* — "HealthGrades is a unique award-winning Internet service that accurately and objectively grades the performance of healthcare providers in the United States. HealthGrades users want to take charge of their healthcare so they come to HealthGrades to find the best healthcare provider. HealthGrades' clients include healthcare providers, employees, health plans, insurance companies and consumers" (www.healthgrades.com).

- *Protect Yourself in the Hospital: Insider Tips for Avoiding Hospital Mistakes for Yourself or Someone You Love* by Thomas A. Sharon

- *Evidence-Based Practice in Nursing & Healthcare*: *A Guide to Best Practice* by B. Melnyk and E. Fineout-Overholt (editors)
- Journal: *Evidence-Based Nursing* by BMJ Publishing Group
- Journal: *Worldviews on Evidence-Based Nursing* by Blackwell Publishing and Sigma Theta Tau International

References

Aydin, C. E., Bolton, L. B., Donaldson, N., Brown, D. S., Buffum, M., Elashoff, J. D. & Sandhu, M. (2004). Creating and analyzing a statewide nursing quality measurement database. *Journal of Nursing Scholarship, 36* (4), 371-378.

Institute for Healthcare Improvement's 100,000 Lives Campaign. Retrieved from www.ihi.org on February 15, 2005.

Institute of Medicine. (2000). *To err is human: Building a safer health system.* Washington, DC: National Academy Press.

Joint Commission on Accreditation of Healthcare Organization's National Patient Safety goals. Retrieved from www.jcaho.org on February 15, 2005.

Patient safety in the news: Overworking nurses has adverse effects on patient safety. Retrieved from www.gvsu.edu on December 12, 2004.

Rosenstein, A. & O'Daniel, M. (2005). Disruptive behavior and clinical outcomes: Perceptions of physicians and nurses. *Nursing Management, 36* (1), 18-27.

The Leapfrog Group for Patient Safety. Retrieved from www.leapfroggroup.org on February 15, 2005.

Chapter Eleven
Mentoring

"Treat people as if they were what they ought to be and you help them become what they are capable of being." — *Eudora Welty, author and photographer* ◆

Nurses have often been accused of "eating their young." This is a phrase we could do without. We need to do a better job of coaching and mentoring each other. We all know that it is very hard to "hang in there" as a seasoned nurse. It is even harder for a new nurse or a nurse new to an environment.

In the role of charge nurse there is plenty of opportunity to coach and mentor. Be a hero. When you are in charge, take time to consider the people who are in need of mentoring. Try to remember what it has been like for you and put yourself in the new person's shoes. Do for them what was done for you (or what you wish had been done for you).

Painful experiences that occur during orientation remain memories for a long time. The first time I passed medications on my first job is one such memory for me. I was partnered with an experienced nurse who was very focused on my progress. This part of the memory is good. I felt that my performance was a priority for her and that she was taking seriously the responsibility of teaching me on the job. On the 8 a.m. medication rounds, I had a "near miss." A patient was scheduled for surgery and I failed to note this. I almost medicated her, but caught the error in time. At the end of the day, the nurse assigned to orient me told me that she thought I had made a mistake in choosing the profession of nursing. She berated me for my inattention to detail and accused me of having an uncaring attitude toward the patients. This was devastating. I will never forget it. The approach worked in that it had the effect of making me determined to come back the next day and do a better job; however, it also left me with a determination to be an encouraging and positive mentor. Learning through fear and intimidation is not usually effective. A good mentor inspires trust and confidence.

It is likely that nearly every day you are in charge you will be given the opportunity to coach and mentor. Brand new nurses, experienced new hires, floats, per diem nurses, new charge nurses, new managers, new people in other departments, residents, fellows and new physicians are some examples. Healthcare organizations hire many people. Every month there is a new batch of protégés. Wouldn't it be great if they stayed with the organization for a long time? It would decrease the shortage of workers and eliminate the feeling that "everyone around here is so new they don't quite know what they are doing."

"I know of no more encouraging fact than the unquestionable ability of man to elevate his life by conscious endeavor."
— *Henry David Thoreau, author, poet and philosopher*

The Cost of Poor Mentoring

It is estimated that organizations spend between $2,000 and $11,000 to hire each employee. This number is even higher for the recruitment of nurses because they are highly skilled professionals and they are scarce. It is also estimated that as many as 50 percent of new hires leave within the first six months *if they do not receive a solid orientation*. It is only at the end of six months that employees are able to be as productive as an experienced worker. It takes even longer than six months for nurses, particularly specialty nurses, to be fully on their own.

So, you can see that a lot of money will be saved when we retain nurses; however, that is not the most important reason to coach, mentor and retain nurses. The *standard of care* in any healthcare organization is directly related to the expertise and tenure of its nurses. Excellent nurses who have worked together over time deliver the best care. Everyone benefits. Patients get better care, physicians have better outcomes, nurses grow more and more excellent and the satisfaction of patients, nurses and physicians improves. The list goes on. It is a win-win for everyone. On the flip side, if excellent nurses are not retained, patient care deteriorates, errors are made, morale is low and the downward spiral of exiting nurses goes on and on.

It seems so easy to understand. It is so logical. And yet, it is difficult to find a healthcare organization where nurse orientation and training is given the high priority it deserves. Strides are being made in this area; healthcare administrators are making changes to correct this. Meanwhile, each of us has to take it on as a challenge and a mission to *nurture our young* and develop great nurses.

"Two hallmarks that distinguish the good mentor from the mediocre teacher are recognition that passion is central to learning and the capacity to provide emotional support when it is needed." — *Stephen Brookfield, educator*

Good Mentoring Takes Time

Wherever you work, it is likely that there is an orientation program. There is probably a plan and a process that is tailored to every protégé. The barrier to carrying out these plans is usually time. It takes a lot of time to do a good job of orienting, coaching and mentoring. The key component is quality time; however, setting aside time for the required communication and documentation is given a low priority in the crunch to get all of the work done each day. It is even sometimes difficult to consistently pair a new nurse with the same person day after day. Schedules and other responsibilities cause the orientation plan to get lost in the shuffle, which may cause the new nurse to feel personally lost, alone and unimportant to the organization and the nurses with whom he or she works.

There is no easy answer. Try to make time. Developing a new nurse is definitely a wonderful way to spend your time. It is the opportunity to transact the passage of the wisdom, caring and confidence you have developed. The most magical thing you can do is to develop a supportive and encouraging relationship with the person you are mentoring.

There is a phenomenon known as the *Pygmalion Effect*. You are probably familiar with it. It is a performance stimulating effect. People who are led to expect that they will do well, will do better than those who expect to do poorly, or do not have any expectations about how well or how poorly they will do. Mentors who arouse in protégés confidence in their abilities will increase the likelihood of protégé success. When a mentor spends time with a protégé and expresses satisfaction, praise and encouragement, the protégé is more likely to do well. A positive, accepting and supportive relationship with a protégé is likely to result in developing a positive, confident and caring nurse.

"My chief want in life is someone who shall make me do what I can." — *Ralph Waldo Emerson, author, poet and philosopher*

Characteristics of a Good Mentor

Experience has shown that the best nursing mentor:

- has a positive attitude
- is a role model
- communicates well
- listens well
- provides moral support, guidance and advice
- performs well under stress
- demonstrates interpersonal problem-solving skills
- demonstrates proficient or expert practice
- is a good resource person
- encourages protégés
- is successful in building caring relationships
- is committed to meeting with protégés on a regular basis
- is good at giving honest and constructive feedback
- is committed to completing the required documentation and evaluation forms

Benefits for the Mentor

Experience has also shown that there are many benefits for the mentor:

- satisfaction and continued learning intrinsic to teaching
- development of professional colleagues
- development of self-awareness
- development of interpersonal relationships
- professional development
- stimulation to question practice

Not everyone likes to orient or train new people. It is hard to do if you are not very experienced or confident in yourself. People who volunteer to be mentors and then receive some training do the best job at mentoring. It is helpful to know not only the steps and forms required in the process, but also how adults learn.

"If learning is about growth, and growth requires both trust and agency, then teaching is about recognizing and nourishing the conditions in which trust and agency can flourish. Teaching is thus preeminently an act of care." — *Larry Daloz, author on teaching and mentoring*

The Complexity of Learning

The process of becoming a new nurse or even of learning a new role in a new environment is complex. Cognitive learning is going on at the same time as socialization. Here is a partial list of the dimensions of learning that occur for every nurse:

- *Autonomy* — advocacy, critical thinking, decision making, application of theory vs. real practice, personal trustworthiness
- *Care Delivery* — care planning, preventing and managing crises, skill performance, task management, time management, assessment and intervention

- *Cultural Adaptation* — finding a fit between personal values and the values of the organization
- *Information Management* — communication, documentation and technology
- *Leadership* — delegation, supervision, motivation and inspiration
- *Psychological Management* — stress, conflict, expectations, tiredness, anxiety, fear, feeling like an outsider, dignity and loneliness
- *Relationship Management* — people, personalities, team dynamics and physicians
- *Adapting to Change* — learning, unlearning and feeling overwhelmed

Every nurse is learning about all of these every day. It is part of being an individual functioning in an organization. For a new nurse, this learning is magnified dramatically. Developing a caring and supportive relationship with a mentor can make all the difference between failing and succeeding.

Be a great mentor. Be a role model. Be a friend. Make the time. Teach by doing. Step back and let them do. Discuss feelings. Build confidence. Create a nurse. Be a hero.

"My continuing passion is to part a curtain, that invisible shadow that falls between people, the veil of indifference to each other's presence, each other's wonder, each other's human plight." — *Eudora Welty, author and photographer*

Making Mentoring Work

Russell and Adams (1997) define mentoring as an "intense interpersonal exchange between a senior experienced colleague (mentor) and a less experienced, junior colleague (protégé) in which the mentor provides support, direction and feedback regarding career plans and personal development" (p. 2). In addition, "mentors are frequently characterized as individuals who are committed to providing support to junior members in an effort to remove organizational barriers and to increase the upward mobility of their protégés" (p. 2).

In their article *Making Mentoring Work*, Tabborn, Macaulay, & Cook (1997) discuss four key factors that make mentoring work: 1) a clear, agreed upon set of objectives; 2) communication and training; 3) matching of mentors and protégés; and 4) evaluation and review of the program. First, the unit needs to have a clear picture of how and why the mentoring program will be utilized. How will the mentoring program assist the unit in meeting its objectives? A clear definition, along with the support of unit mentors, will form a solid foundation for the program. Second, unit leaders will need education on the process of mentoring and they will need a clear understanding of their role in the process. What are their objectives and expectations? What is their time commitment? All of these questions need to be answered. Further, mentors should be briefed (at least) in techniques of active listening, facilitation and base-line skill building. Third, the process for matching mentors with protégés should be thought through in a careful manner. There are a number of methods, and no one process has an overarching stamp of approval. Regardless of the process, the unit should be aware of how the method will affect mentors as well as protégés. Finally, units must evaluate and review their progress. Not only will this process assist the unit in determining success of the program, it will also assist unit leaders in evaluating the effect on the protégé.

Case Study – Mentoring

Mentoring on your unit has always been a bit of a joke. In fact, everyone jokes about it — even the doctors. Maybe it's because mentoring is regarded as a mandate from administration. Maybe it's because everyone is so busy that it is "just one more thing." Maybe it is because no one sees any value in it. Who knows? You have been a charge nurse for five years and have the respect of your team. You just talked with a friend, Sarah, at Central University Hospital who spoke very highly of its mentoring program. In fact, she sent along some materials about the program and how it is designed. It looks *really* good and you see how it could benefit your unit.

You go home excited and think about how this program could work on your unit. You know you would probably have the buy-in of your supervisor but you think that you would *not* have the buy-in of your unit colleagues. Sarah's materials look good, but you know you can take it to the next level. You begin to develop a plan for your unit.

- What is successful about the mentoring program on your unit?
- What aspects are not successful?
- What barriers are getting in the way of a successful program?
- Who is involved in mentoring? Do they want to be mentors?
- Do they receive education on how to be mentors?
- Are they recognized for their efforts?
- How long does the mentoring program last?
- Are clear expectations written for mentors and protégés?
- You know some will view your ideas for this program as *one more thing.* How will you sell it to your supervisor and your colleagues?
- Who else should be included in planning?

Reflections

- Who are the individuals in your life that have had a large impact on your progress?
- What was it about these individuals that helped you along the way?
- What do you think are the most important attributes of a mentor?
- Have you ever been a mentor? To whom? Were you effective as a mentor? Why or why not?

- How does the mentoring system on your unit work? Is it an effective system or does it need improvement? What changes are needed to improve it?
- Are you a mentor as a charge nurse? Formal or informal?
- What is the vacancy rate for RNs in your healthcare organization? In your opinion, is this a reflection of the mentoring process in your healthcare organization?

Remember...

- Mentoring is one of the most important roles an individual can play within a unit. Helping someone to acclimate to co-workers and equipment is an important role because it defines and shapes a new team member's initial impressions of the unit and of the organization. It may leave them thinking, "This is uncomfortable" *or* "This is where I want to work."
- Structure your mentoring program in a way that everything is spelled out. What are the expectations of the mentor? How about the protégé? How long will the relationship last?
- Who is your mentor? If the process does not exist formally within your healthcare organization, seek someone you respect and ask them if they would like to have lunch once a month. According to Scandura, *et al.* (1996), research has shown that protégé promotions and compensation appear to be influenced by a mentor. Moreover, Forret *et al.* (1996) note that mentors provide protégés with career functions such as how to maneuver organizational politics, etc. They also provide protégés with psychosocial functions which increase their competence, effectiveness and work-role identity. Give yourself a gift and find a mentor!
- Good mentoring relationships are built on trust, allowing protégés the opportunity to build confidence in the process. Choose mentors who will take this commitment seriously.

Additional Resources on Mentoring

- *Mentoring: How to Develop Successful Mentor Behaviors* by Gordon F. Shea
- *A Mentor's Companion* by Larry Ambrose
- *Woman to Woman: Preparing Yourself to Mentor* by Edna Ellison & Tricia Scribner
- *The Mentor Connection in Nursing* by Connie Vance & Roberta K. Olson

References

Bass, B. (1985). *Leadership and performance beyond expectations.* New York: Free Press.

Forret, et al. (1996). Issues facing organizations when implementing formal mentoring programmes. *Leadership and Organization Development Journal, 17* (3), 27-30.

Mullich, M. (2004). They're hired: Now the real recruiting begins. Workforce Management OnLine, January, 2004. Retrieved from www.workforce.com on January 12, 2005.

Reeves, K.A. (2004). Nurses nurturing nurses: A mentoring program. *Nurse Leader, 2* (6), 47-49.

Russell, J. & Adams, D. (1997). The changing nature of mentoring in organizations: An introduction to the special issue on mentoring in organizations. *Journal of Vocational Behaviors, 51,* 1-14.

Scandura, et al. (1996). Perspectives on mentoring. *Leadership and Organization Development Journal, 17* (3), 50-56.

Squires, A. (2004). A dimensional analysis of role enactment of acute care nurses. *Journal of Nursing Scholarship, 36* (3), 272-278.

Tabborn, A., Macaulay, S., & Cook, S. (1997). *Making mentoring work. Training for Quality, 5* (1), 6-9.

Chapter Twelve
Remember your Mission

It seems like this would go without saying.

You are there for the patient. You are there to make sure the patient receives the very best care possible and, in your role as charge nurse, you do much of this through other people. Therefore, you are there to be the best leader possible. Through your skillful management and guidance, your mission is to motivate the healthcare team to give the patient the very best health care possible.

While it may seem obvious, reminding yourself that you are here for the patients is essential. The team should remember that as well. The world in which our work is done is so busy, stressful, fast-paced and full of competing priorities that sometimes the reason for our work gets lost. We are only human and yet our work demands us — and we demand of ourselves — to be superhuman. It is so easy to get off track — to get discouraged, become frustrated and let ourselves down.

"The sheer act of love transcends the outcome." — *Mother Teresa, spiritual leader*

One day I was called by a physician from his car. It was early in the morning and he was visiting all of his patients in various community hospitals before he opened for office hours. He was trying to be in several places at once. He asked if I would bring all of his patients' charts to the front desk so that he could make entries in them without having to actually make rounds. *He had forgotten his mission.* We talked for a few minutes about how much his patients were looking forward to seeing him. He realized without having to say it out loud how far he had strayed from his purpose. He made rounds. He got back on track.

"It is the nature of man to rise to greatness if greatness is expected of him." — *John Steinbeck, author*

Here is another example: When I was a hospital executive at the beginning of each year every department sent me their goals and action plans for the year. One year, I received a plan from a support department. The employees in this department were not responsible for direct patient care; however, through their daily work they supported direct patient caregivers. As I read their goals and action plans for the year, I realized that nowhere in the document had they used the word *patient*. It was evident that serving the patient was implied, but it was not directly stated. I sent the document back for revision. It was a good department. They did their work well, but I felt it was important that they remember their mission by including the word patient in their annual plan of work.

"Technological improvements do not do away with the importance of having that link with an individual, that response from another being, which is what nursing perhaps defines most clearly." — *Queen Elizabeth II of England*

Stay on Track

Remember to stay on track. It is good to stop and reflect upon where you are in relation to your mission. Why did you become a nurse in the first place? Why did you choose this profession as your life's work? Do you remember your first clinical rotation? Do you remember that feeling of eagerness to be a nurse someday? Do you remember the day you passed your state board examination? Do you remember your first day on the job? Can you believe how much you have learned and grown since then?

It is good to reflect upon where you have come from and where you are going. It is helpful to think about where you are today compared with where you aspire to be. It is motivating to have goals and to work toward them and, once they are achieved, to set new goals that cause you to grow and stretch even more. You will find strength and inspiration in understanding the gap between the realities of who you are now and the vision of who you want to be.

"Nurses know how to listen, how to reach out, how to respect."
— *Comelio Sommaruga, President, International Committee of the Red Cross*

Your Personal Mission Statement

You are the only one who knows your personal mission. Take some time to think about it. What is your mission each day? Each year? For your life? Writing down your personal mission, values and goals is a worthwhile exercise. Doing so helps you think about what is important to you and what you want to accomplish. Read it once a month and ask yourself: Am I on track? Am I proud of the person I see in the mirror? Are the people I care about proud of me? Am I the kind of adult I dreamed about being when I was a child? Am I living up to my potential? Am I being all I can be? Am I taking care of myself?

A written mission or vision is a powerful thing. A shortened version can become a daily mantra to help you stay on track. We nurses have a tendency to reflect negatively upon our work — we dwell on what we did not get done, and what we should have done; which often happens to nurses in their thoughts on the way home from work. Replace those self-deprecating thoughts with positive thoughts "I did a lot of good today. I made a positive difference in many lives." You have to fill up the well of giving to keep on giving.

It is your mission, too, to represent the nursing profession. Now and then, a poll is done by Gallup or some other group in the business of gathering information from the public, to survey the public perception of various professional groups. Almost always, nurses come out at the very top or near the very top as being honest, ethical and trusted. The public has a very high opinion of nurses. It is the responsibility of each of us to live up to that reputation. We know from patient satisfaction surveys that nurses are valued highly for their ability to balance competency and technical know-how with caring and compassion. Nurses are beloved for their skills at listening, teaching and communicating.

As a charge nurse you must remember to allow team members the time for the subjective qualities of nursing (e.g., holding a patient's hand for a few minutes or listening to a patient's stories about family). These activities take time away from doing tasks, but they are so very important in fulfilling our mission as nurses.

"To lead people, walk beside them...As for the best leaders, the people do not notice their existence. The next best, the people honor and praise, the next best the people fear, and the next, the people hate...When the best leader's work is done the people say, 'We did it ourselves!'" — *Lau-Tzu, Chinese philosopher*

Nursing requires the qualities sought after by the lion, the scarecrow and the tin man in *The Wizard of Oz*. Courage, Brains and Heart. Risk-taking, intelligent thinking, and loving. Are these concepts part of your personal mission statement?

It is our mission to bring to each other and to our patients, feelings of hope, confidence and inspiration. We need to be mindful of the greater meaning of our work and the effect that it has on our fellow man.

Just before his death in 1963, the great American poet Robert Frost wrote his last poem to his nurse, Janet Forbes: "*I met you on a cloudy and dark day and when you smiled and spoke the room was filled with sunshine. The way you smiled at me has given my heart a change of mood and saved some part of a day I had rued.*"

You are the symbol of hope and comfort and caring. Go forth and light up the world.

Mission Defined

A personal mission statement will answer three primary questions:

- What is the purpose of my life?
- What values do I hold dear?
- What do those values look like in action?

An acute sense of your *values in action* is the most important piece. Once your personal mission statement is written, you need to reflect on how you are doing. You need to revisit it when you are down. You need to share it with others so they can help you. You need to make it a part of your life. Otherwise, it will be words on paper, in a notebook on a shelf, and not "living" and guiding you.

Another way to think about your personal mission is to imagine the following scenario: you are retiring tomorrow and the nurses on your unit are each responsible for saying something about you in front of the group. They have taken truth serum and will offer their honest thoughts. If this were in fact tomorrow, what would they say? What are their perceptions of you and your work? Would they see you as you see yourself as outlined in your mission statement? Answering these questions in an honest fashion can give you a rough idea of how your role as charge nurse aligns with your personal mission statement.

Remember...

- In his song, *Any Road*, George Harrison of The Beatles wrote, "If you don't know where you're going, any road will take you there." A mission statement is a personal roadmap that can always help you find your way. No matter what roads those around you are on, you always know where you are headed. Give yourself this gift and then make it live.

- Take a close look at your organization's mission and place it next to your own mission. How well do they align?
- Keep in mind that, like you, at times your organization will struggle with living up to its mission...what a wonderful opportunity and what valuable work to help it realign!
- You must remember to stay on track. It is good to stop and reflect upon where you are in relation to your mission. Why did you become a nurse in the first place? Why did you choose this profession as your life's work? Do you remember your first clinical rotation? Do you remember that feeling of eagerness to be a nurse someday? Do you remember the day you passed your state board examination? Do you remember your first day on the job? Can you believe how much you have learned and grown since that day?
- Nursing takes the qualities sought after by the lion, the scarecrow and the tin man in *The Wizard of Oz*. Courage, Brains and Heart.

Additional Resources

- *The Path: Creating Your Mission Statement for Work and for Life* by Laurie Beth Jones
- *Character Is Destiny: The Value of Personal Ethics in Everyday Life* by Russell Gough

References

Frost, R. (n.d.). *Miss Forbes*. Quoted in an article by Klein, J. (2002). Teaching palliative care and education. *Oncology Times*, 24 (12), 79-80.

Hitti, M. (2004). Nurses Top List for Honesty. Retrieved from http://webcenter.health.webmd/ on December 29, 2004.

Contact the Authors
Today!

We would love to hear from you! How can we improve this book? What stories would you like to share? What should we include in future editions?

Cathy Leary and Scott Allen may be contacted for inquires, speaking engagements, workshops and interviews as follows:

Cathy Leary, R.N.
Phone: 440-285-8788
Email: cathy@cldmail.com

Scott J. Allen, Ph.D.
Phone: 216-224-7072
Email: scott@cldmail.com

Order Information

To order copies of this publication, contact BookMasters at:

Phone: 800-247-6553
Fax: 419-281-6883
Email: orders@bookmasters.com
Web: www.atlasbooks.com
Mail: BookMasters Inc.
          30 Amberwood Parkway
          Ashland, Ohio 44805